THE EMPOWERED NEW MOM

A PARENT'S GUIDE TO RAISING HAPPY, HEALTHY, AND CONFIDENT CHILDREN FROM NEWBORN TO TODDLERHOOD

SARA LYLES

Preface

The act of bearing and raising babies is commonly perceived as one of the most natural things in the world. Regardless of their background and education, all mothers possess certain instincts and compassion that enable them to care for their children. However, as life becomes more complicated and medical science continues to evolve, mothers face new challenges in raising their children. Mothers need to learn about the best ways to raise their children, protect them from illnesses, and interact with them in ways that promote self-confidence, discipline, faith, moral values, and sound ethics.

This book provides an in-depth overview of the mother's role in the first four years of a child's life. It sheds light on various important issues that parents must pay attention to as they raise their children. The author provides practical advice and strategies to help new mothers navigate child-rearing challenges. Moreover, the book highlights some traditional child-rearing practices that can harm a child's well-being and suggests more beneficial alternatives.

By following the guidelines in this book, new mothers can raise a balanced child who will be an asset to themselves, their families, and society at large.

Table of Contents

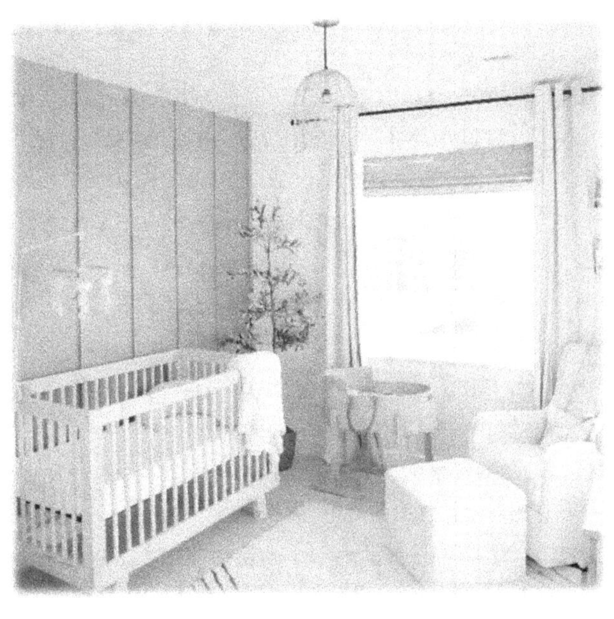

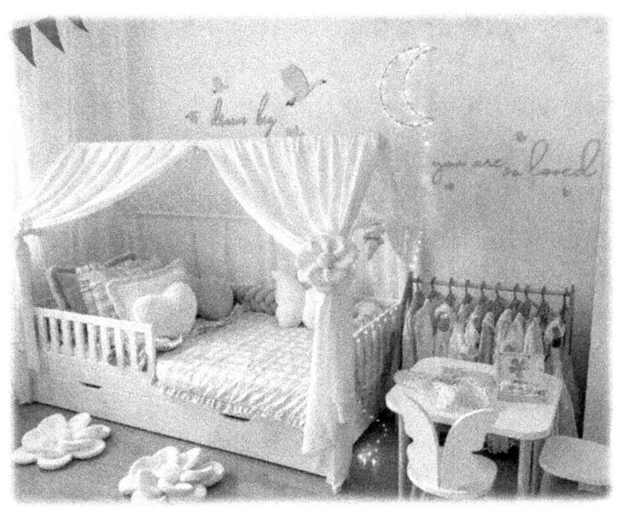

INTRODUCTION

Dear mother,

I would like to congratulate you on the arrival or expected arrival of your new baby. As we live in an era of rapid changes and developments, it is essential to prepare thoroughly for the arrival of your little one. Raising a child who can keep up with the latest developments and challenges is crucial. To ensure your child is well-equipped, you must be aware of everything related to caring for your child from birth through the various stages of development.

It is important to understand what each stage of your child's development requires based on modern theories and research in many fields. This includes understanding your baby's nutritional requirements, how to keep them clean, how to dress them, how to put them to sleep, what to do when they cry, and the various activities they may engage in as they grow.

To make things easier for you, a book has been written to answer all your questions about taking care of yourself after giving birth and everything you need to take care of your baby. The book covers nutrition, cleanliness, dressing, sleep, crying, growth, development, and various activities. The book also includes sections on child health, sickness, and how to deal with accidents (first aid).

These topics have been presented simply and straightforwardly for all mothers. I hope this book will benefit all mothers and fathers, helping them raise a generation that will restore humanity's glory. As a Japanese thinker once said, most nations of the world live on resources that lie beneath their feet, which will run out with the passage of time. Therefore, raising children who can adapt to the changes and challenges that the world throws their way is crucial.

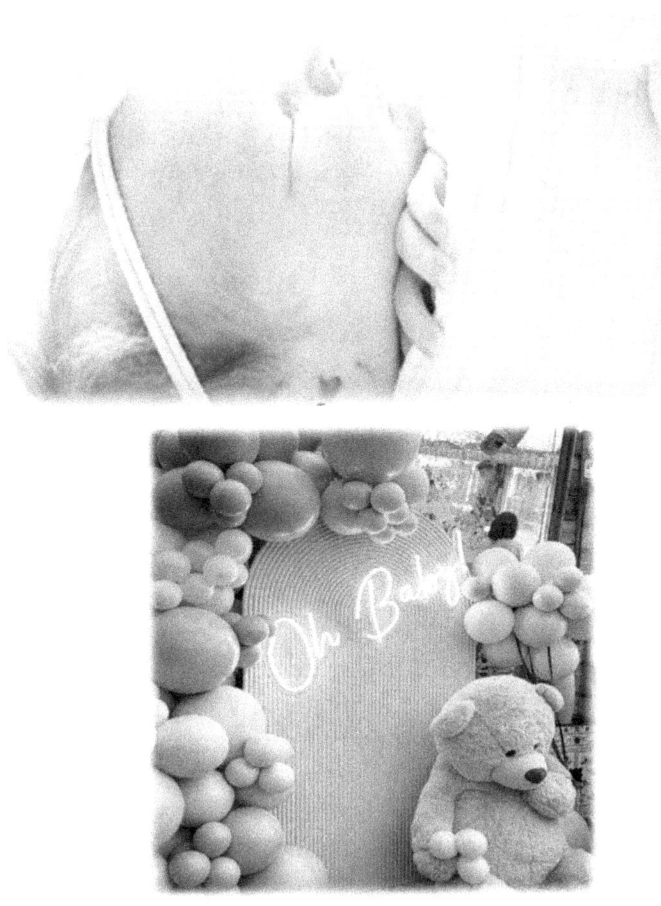

CHAPTER ONE

Preparing to welcome the newborn

Preparing for a new baby involves many important tasks. Below is a guide to some of the essential things you'll need to take care of before the baby arrives.

Setting up the nursery

To create a comfortable sleeping space for your baby, you'll need essentials like a bassinet or crib, sheets, and blankets. You might also consider adding decorative items to personalize the nursery.

Essential clothing and supplies for the baby

- 6 sleep suits
- 6 undershirts (ones that fasten between the baby's legs)
- Bibs
- Socks (if sleep suits have feet, socks may not be necessary)
- Coat or "snowsuit" for cold weather
- 3-4 sets of clothes for going out
- 2 receiving blankets (for swaddling, burping, etc.)
- Woolen blankets, especially for winter

When buying supplies, consider the season in which your baby will be born to avoid purchasing clothes unsuitable for the weather. Also, ensure the clothing fabric is comfortable for your baby's skin, avoiding materials that may cause itching. Cotton, cotton blends, and knit fabrics are usually the most comfortable options.

Hygiene practices for newborn care

- 6-8 packets of diapers in various sizes
- Sterilized cotton gauze for cleaning the baby's belly button
- Soap and shampoo suitable for newborns
- Diaper rash cream
- Wet wipes for baby's hygiene
- Plastic bags for dirty diapers
- Soft towels for drying after baths
- Soft comb and brush for gentle grooming
- Safety scissors with rounded ends for nail trimming
- Baby bathtub for bathing ease

Feeding options and considerations

If you plan to breastfeed, you might consider purchasing a breast pump to extract milk and sterilized plastic bottles to store the milk.

Getting around with the baby

You'll need an infant car seat, a pram or stroller, and a baby carrier or sling to ensure your baby's safety and convenience. These essentials will help you transport your baby comfortably and securely, whether in the car, walking, or running errands.

Here's what to expect in terms of your newborn's appearance:

- Your baby may have a large head with no noticeable neck, short legs, and a large torso.
- The head of most newborns might look somewhat distorted due to being squeezed in the birth canal for an average of twelve hours during delivery. Babies born via Cesarean section often have a different appearance since their heads haven't experienced the same compression.
- Don't worry about the soft spot on your baby's skull, called the fontanelle, which allows for passage through the birth canal. The rear part typically closes within about 4 months, while the front part may take between nine and eighteen months to close completely.
- Your baby may also have some swelling in the genital area due to the extra dose of female hormones received just before birth. Additionally, their face and eyes may appear swollen, lips may be rosy, and hands and feet may have a bluish tint in the first few hours of life.

your baby's first cry

When your baby cries for the first time, it shows that their breathing system works well. This cry means they're now breathing air instead of getting oxygen from the placenta. It also tells us that their airways are clear, and there are no problems with their voice or breathing. Any changes in their cry could mean something needs attention.

Your baby's skin

The infant's skin is naturally coated with a smooth, white, waxy substance called vernix. Its purpose is to safeguard the baby's skin from rashes during the initial days after birth, gradually being absorbed by the body over time.

Concerns about blue spots, known as "Mongolian blue spots," on the skin are unnecessary. These spots, typically found in children with darker skin tones, are unrelated to bruises or circulation issues. However, if the spots appear red, it could indicate pores not functioning optimally or pressure during birth. Fortunately, these red spots usually fade within a week or ten days after birth.

Your baby's Hair

Upon birth, the child's Hair is typically soft and dark, but it will shed within the first week, allowing new hair growth. Additionally, you may notice fine Hair covering various parts of the baby's body, like the cheeks, ears, shoulders, and back, which usually disappears by the fourth month.

It's important to note that the appearance of the baby's Hair at birth doesn't predict its future characteristics. Babies born with little or no Hair may eventually develop blond Hair, while those with blond Hair at birth might see it darken over time. Your baby's hair color may not be apparent at birth, and it might take some time before you can determine its true color.

Your baby's eye

After birth, it's common for the baby's eyes to appear swollen due to pressure during delivery, but this typically resolves quickly. Additionally, you may notice a yellowish substance in the eyes, which could result from a blocked tear duct or a minor eye infection. Your doctor can prescribe drops to treat this issue if necessary.

Eye color

The true color of the baby's eyes may not become apparent until they are a few months old. The initial color they have right after birth may change as the child develops and their body produces melanin, which affects eye color. Although rare, it's also possible for a child to be born with eyes of different colors.

It's common for a baby's nose to be blocked, so avoid using nose drops or other remedies without consulting a doctor first. A white tongue is natural since the baby relies solely on milk for nourishment. However, if you notice white spots on a pink tongue, it could indicate thrush, an overgrowth of yeast in the baby's mouth. Your doctor can provide guidance on appropriate treatment in such cases.

Identifying and managing common concerns like jaundice

Infant jaundice is characterized by yellowish discoloration of a newborn's skin and eyes, caused by an excess of bilirubin in the blood. This condition is common, especially in preterm babies and some breastfed infants, as their livers may not yet be fully developed to efficiently process bilirubin. While most babies born between 35 weeks' gestation and a full term typically do not require treatment for jaundice, in rare cases, elevated bilirubin levels can pose a risk of brain damage, particularly when specific risk factors are present. Early detection and monitoring are crucial to ensure the baby's well-being.

Symptoms

The primary sign of infant jaundice is the yellowing of the skin and the whites of the eyes, typically appearing between the second and fourth day after birth.

To check for jaundice, gently press on your baby's forehead or nose. If the skin appears yellow when you press, it may indicate mild jaundice. In contrast, if your baby doesn't have jaundice, the skin color should return to its normal shade after pressing.

Ensure you examine your baby in well-lit conditions, preferably natural daylight, to assess their skin color accurately. Early detection is essential for timely management of jaundice.

When to see a doctor

Most hospitals have a protocol for checking newborns for jaundice before discharge. The American Academy of Pediatrics advises parents to ensure their newborn babies undergo routine checks for jaundice during medical exams and at least every 8 to 12 hours while in the hospital. It is important to have your baby examined for jaundice between the third and seventh day after birth when bilirubin levels typically reach their peak. If your baby is discharged within 72 hours after birth, schedule a follow-up appointment for a jaundice check within two days of discharge.

Be vigilant for signs of severe jaundice or complications from excess bilirubin. Contact your doctor if you notice:

- Increasing yellowing of your baby's skin
- Yellowing of the abdomen, arms, or legs
- The whites of your baby's eyes turning yellow
- Lethargy or difficulty waking your baby
- Poor weight gain or feeding difficulties

- High-pitched crying or other concerning symptoms

Prompt medical attention is crucial if you observe any of these signs or symptoms in your baby.

Causes

Jaundice is primarily caused by excess bilirubin (hyperbilirubinemia). Bilirubin, responsible for the yellow hue of jaundice, is a natural byproduct of the breakdown of red blood cells.

Newborns tend to produce more bilirubin than adults due to increased red blood cell breakdown in the first days of life. While the liver normally filters bilirubin from the bloodstream, releasing it into the intestines, a newborn's immature liver may struggle to process bilirubin efficiently, accumulating bilirubin in the body. This common occurrence, physiologic jaundice, typically manifests on the second or third day after birth.

Other causes

While physiologic jaundice is common and typically occurs in newborns due to the liver's temporary inability to efficiently process bilirubin, jaundice can also result from underlying disorders. In these cases, jaundice may manifest earlier or later than usual.

Conditions that can lead to jaundice in infants include:

- Internal bleeding (hemorrhage)
- Blood infection (sepsis)
- Other viral or bacterial infections

- Blood type incompatibility between mother and baby
- Liver dysfunction
- Biliary atresia, a blockage or scarring of the bile ducts
- Enzyme deficiencies
- Abnormalities in red blood cells causing rapid breakdown

If your baby develops jaundice outside the typical timeframe or shows signs of jaundice-related complications, prompt medical attention is essential for proper diagnosis and management.

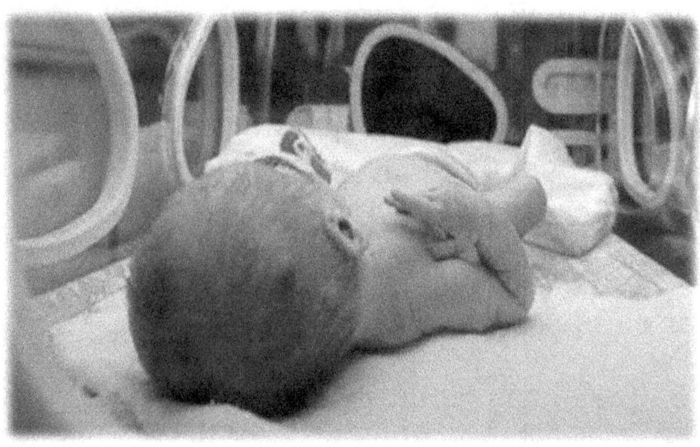

Prevention

Adequate feeding is the best preventive measure against infant jaundice. For breastfed infants, aim for 8 to 12 daily feedings during the first few days of life. Formula-fed infants typically require 1 to 2 ounces (about 30 to 60 milliliters) of formula every two to three hours during the first week.

Consistent feeding helps ensure the baby receives enough nutrition to support healthy liver function and bilirubin processing, reducing the risk of jaundice.

Vaccination

Many countries follow a vaccination schedule that includes administering a sequence of vaccines at specific stages of a child's growth, usually starting from birth. While mandatory in some countries, these schedules are suggested in others. Below, you can find a table that outlines the primary vaccinations included in such schedules.

Age at vaccination	Vaccine
At birth	Tuberculosis (TB) Hepatitis B
At 2 months	Poliomyelitis (polio) Hepatitis B DPT (diphtheria, pertussis (whooping cough) and tetanus) Pneumococcal
At 4 months	Poliomyelitis (polio) Hepatitis B DPT (diphtheria, Pertussis (whooping cough) and Tetanus) Pneumococcal
At 6 months	Poliomyelitis (polio) Hepatitis B

	DPT (diphtheria, Pertussis (whooping cough) and Tetanus) Pneumococcal
At 12 months	Poliomyelitis (polio)
At 18 months	Poliomyelitis (polio) DPT (diphtheria, Pertussis (whooping cough) and Tetanus) Pneumococcal Hepatitis A
At 24 months	Hepatitis A
At 4-6 years	Poliomyelitis (polio) DPT (diphtheria, Pertussis (whooping cough) and Tetanus) MMR (measles, mumps, rubella) Varicella (chicken pox)

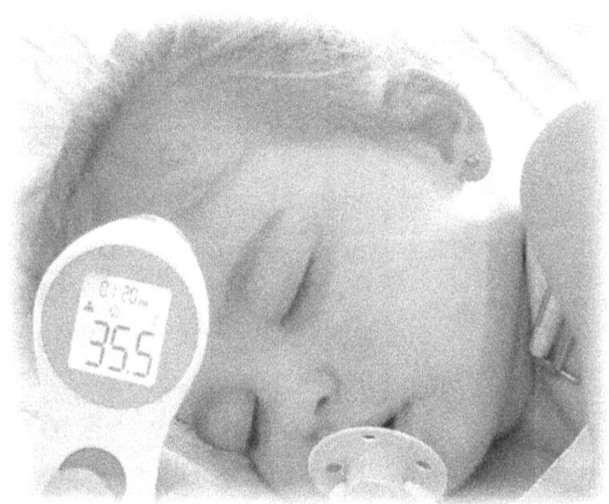

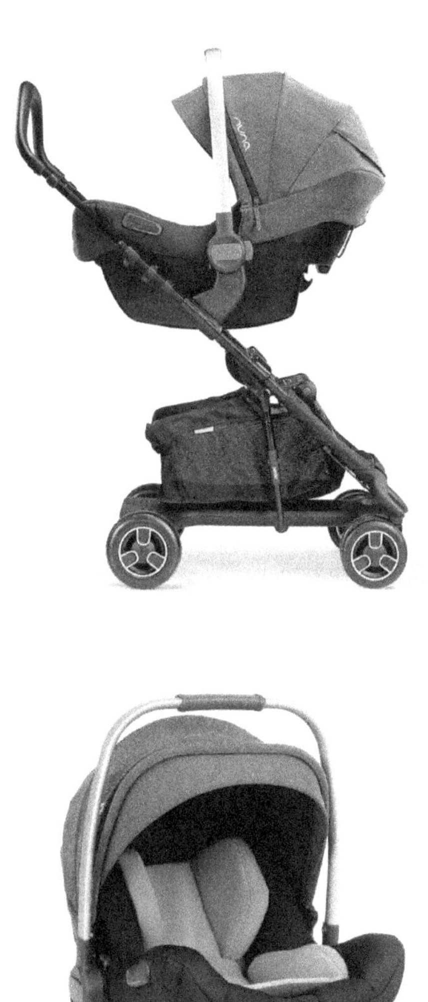

Baby shower

What is a Baby Shower?
A baby shower is a celebration to honor a pregnant mother and welcome her new arrival. It's a time for friends and family to gather, share well wishes, and offer gifts to help the mother prepare for her baby's arrival.

Who Hosts the Baby Shower?
Traditionally, a close friend or family member hosts the baby shower. Still, nowadays, it's not uncommon for multiple people to co-host or for the expectant mother to be involved in the planning.

When to Have the Baby Shower?
Baby showers are typically held during the later stages of pregnancy, usually in the third trimester, to ensure that the mother is comfortable and the baby's gender is known, if applicable.

Invitations
Invitations should be sent about four to six weeks before the baby shower.

Include important details such as the date, time, location, RSVP information, and any special requests or themes.

Themes and Decorations

Selecting a particular theme for the baby shower can be an enjoyable and effective way to add a fun and cohesive element to the event. Common themes include animals, books, colors, or nursery rhymes. Decorations such as balloons, banners, and table settings can complement the theme and create a festive atmosphere.

Games and Activities

Baby shower games and activities are a great way to break the ice and keep guests entertained. Popular games include guessing the baby's birth date, diaper-changing races, and baby item memory games.

Gifts

Guests typically bring gifts for the expectant mother and baby. Common gifts include clothing, diapers, baby gear, and nursery essentials. It's helpful to include a registry with the invitations to guide guests in their gift selections.

Food and Refreshments

Refreshments are an important part of any baby shower. Consider serving finger foods, appetizers, and desserts to accommodate guests' tastes. Non-alcoholic beverages such as punch, lemonade, or mocktails are suitable options for refreshments.

Thank You Notes

After the baby shower, the expectant mother should send thank you notes to express gratitude for the gifts and support received. Personalized notes are thoughtful and show appreciation for the guests' generosity.

Enjoy the Celebration

Above all, remember that the baby shower is a time to celebrate the expectant mother and her new arrival. Enjoy the festivities, cherish the memories made, and look forward to welcoming the newest family member!

Circumcision considerations and cultural perspectives

Circumcision is a surgical procedure aimed at removing the foreskin, the skin covering the tip of the penis. It holds significance in various cultures as a religious or ceremonial tradition, notably within Jewish and Islamic faiths. In the United States, newborn circumcision is elective, with approximately 64 percent of newborn boys undergoing the procedure, although rates vary across different socioeconomic, ethnic, and geographic groups.

The decision to circumcise your child is deeply personal and involves considerations of personal beliefs, cultural practices, and religious beliefs, along with potential medical aspects.

While circumcision can be performed at any age, it is commonly done soon after birth or within the first month of life. Local anesthesia is typically used to numb the area during the procedure, and it is often performed while the baby is awake. For older infants, anesthesia is recommended to minimize pain and reduce the risk of injury to the penis. As children grow older, they may become more aware of their bodies, leading to potential psychological impacts associated with the surgery, including fear and anxiety.

What are the potential benefits of circumcision?
If your baby undergoes circumcision, it can simplify penile hygiene for parents and the child, thereby reducing the risk of bacterial infections. Additionally, potential benefits may include:

1. Significantly reduced risk of penile cancer throughout life.
2. Over 90 percent reduction in the risk of urinary tract infections (UTIs) during infancy.
3. Decreased incidence of balanitis (infection of the glands or head of the penis) and posthitis (infection of the prepuce).
4. Prevention of phimosis (inability to retract the foreskin).

Many researchers acknowledge that circumcised men are generally less likely to acquire and transmit HIV and certain sexually transmitted diseases. However, if your child is not circumcised, proper hygiene practices, such as learning to retract the foreskin around the time of toilet training and maintaining cleanliness with daily soap and water, can also be effective in promoting penile health.

Is it a common practice?

Circumcision is indeed widespread. Recent data from the Centers for Disease Control and Prevention (CDC) indicates that the national rate of newborn circumcision in the U.S. is around 60 percent. The data also shows regional variations, with circumcision rates highest in the Midwest and Northeast regions and lowest in the West.

FAQs about circumcision

How old should my child be for circumcision?

Circumcision is a procedure that can be performed at any age, but it is typically done soon after birth or within the first month of life. To mitigate pain during the procedure, a local anesthetic is administered to numb the area, and the surgery is conducted while the baby is awake.

For older infants, anesthesia is recommended to reduce pain and the risk of injury to the penis. As children grow older, they become more conscious of their bodies, leading to increased psychological impacts associated with the surgery, including fear and anxiety.

What are the risks associated with the procedure?

The reported rate of surgical complications for circumcision is relatively low, ranging between 2 to 3 percent, with most being minor instances of postoperative bleeding.

The most common complication involves inadequate removal of the foreskin, prompting parents to request a revision surgery. Serious or life-threatening complications such as penile damage or significant bleeding are exceedingly rare.

However, if your baby has existing heart or lung issues or a bleeding disorder, circumcision may pose risks and should be postponed. Certain congenital conditions may also necessitate more extensive repairs.

Circumcision should be delayed if there are abnormalities such as the urethral opening not being at the tip of the penis, significant curvature of the penis, or if the penis is notably small. It is crucial to consult with a pediatrician to assess the suitability and timing of circumcision for your son, taking into account individual health considerations.

How is circumcision performed?

During circumcision, newborns are typically held still or placed into a circumcision brace to ensure stability. The baby may be comforted, and a local anesthetic may be administered to minimize discomfort.

A protective device is used to remove the skin covering the tip of the penis, followed by the application of gauze with petroleum jelly or antibiotic ointment.

For older children and adults, the procedure is often conducted under general anesthesia to ensure their comfort and safety.

Is it extremely painful for the child?

Contrary to popular belief, circumcision is not typically an extremely painful procedure, especially when local anesthesia is administered. The child may feel pressure and movement with local anesthesia but not pain. The discomfort is minimal, and the child may briefly feel upset while held in place. If the circumcision is conducted under general anesthesia, the child will not experience any pain during the procedure.

Following the procedure, the child should not experience pain during urination, as the urethra, the urinary tube from the bladder through the penis, remains unaffected by circumcision.

What is the recovery process?

Newborns and infants typically recover swiftly from circumcision, often within 12 to 24 hours. Young children typically recover within one to two days, while older children and young adults may take three to four days to recover fully.

After circumcision, temporary skin bruising or mild swelling may occur, which can last for several weeks. These symptoms are usually mild and resolve on their own with time.

Taking care of your child after circumcision

Follow your doctor's guidance, but some general suggestions include:

1. Providing your child with plenty of cuddles and comfort.
2. Apply a small amount of petroleum jelly or ointment to the wound on a light gauze dressing.
3. Applying fresh petroleum jelly and a new gauze dressing at each diaper change to reduce the risk of urine irritation.
4. Give your child a daily bath to keep the area clean.

Physical and emotional changes after childbirth

Immediately after giving birth, you will enter a stage known as postpartum, which typically lasts for about 40 days. During this period, the mother undergoes various physiological changes that gradually restore her body and reproductive organs to their pre-pregnancy state. These changes include the following:

Slight increase in body temperature

This is a natural occurrence resulting from the significant muscular exertion during childbirth, particularly for first-time mothers. This heightened temperature usually lasts for about twenty-four hours. If it persists beyond this timeframe, it could indicate vascular congestion in the breasts or blood in the uterus due to inadequate uterine cleansing, or it may be indicative of puerperal fever, also known as puerperal infection.

Slower than normal heartbeat

This natural phenomenon occurs after childbirth, usually lasting for approximately two or three days. However, if the heartbeat becomes more rapid following birth, it may indicate bleeding or heart disease. Therefore, if there is an increase in the heart rate, it is essential to consult with your obstetrician.

Difficulty in urinating and defecating

These issues may arise from soreness following childbirth or stitches in the case of an episiotomy or tear, which can lead to some discomfort during urination. Alternatively, it could result from the relaxation of the urethra muscles due to pressure from the fetus before and during childbirth. Regarding wounds and minor tears, they typically heal rapidly.

Changes in the uterus

The uterus undergoes a rapid size reduction and returns to its normal state post-birth. This contraction process may be accompanied by some discomfort, particularly after subsequent births, resembling labor pains. These contractions facilitate the expulsion of any remaining pregnancy remnants, usually a mixture of blood and membranes. This expulsion often occurs during breastfeeding, as it triggers the release of hormones that stimulate uterine contraction and shrinkage.

Breastfeeding accelerates the uterus's return to its pre-pregnancy size and weight within about six weeks post-birth. This is because breastfeeding stimulates the breasts, prompting the pituitary gland to release two hormones, prolactin, and oxytocin, which aid in uterine contraction.

Vaginal discharge (lochia)

The discharge color changes throughout the postpartum period. Initially, it's dark red in the first week, transitioning to yellow in the second week, and eventually becoming white by the third week.

The majority of this discharge occurs during the first week after childbirth.

Your stomach may be flabby and not firm.

Your waist circumference might not have fully settled yet, as you may still be shedding the weight gained during pregnancy. Additionally, you might continue to experience back pain and hemorrhoids. Stretch marks may also appear on your chest, stomach, and thighs, particularly if you gained weight rapidly during pregnancy.

If you have undergone a cesarean section

You'll likely feel pain and have difficulty sitting, getting out of bed, standing straight, or walking. However, wounds and small tears should heal quickly.

Self-care tips for new mothers

1. Limit the number of visitors to reduce the risk of exposing the mother to colds or other illnesses.
2. If the weather is warm, the mother should take a warm bath immediately after giving birth.
3. Rest is crucial. The mother should stay in bed during the first few days after birth, gradually increase activity during the second week, and return to bed as needed. By the third week, she can start doing light tasks.

4. Avoid marital relations for forty days to prevent contamination and the entry of germs into the uterus.
5. Pay attention to nutrition to replenish lost blood and increase milk production. A balanced diet with essential nutrients like animal protein, liquids, vitamins, minerals, and energy-rich foods is essential. Avoid foods that cause bloating, such as garlic, onions, and leeks.
6. Regularly consult with the doctor to ensure a smooth recovery during the postpartum period and that the body is returning to its pre-pregnancy state.

Recovering from childbirth and C-section

After a Cesarean birth, the mother requires extra care and complete rest during the initial days.

- In the first twenty-four hours, she may feel dizzy and breathless; she should move slowly.
- Painkillers are necessary if she experiences any pain after the Cesarean, but they should be compatible with breastfeeding.
- The hospital stay typically ranges from three to five days without complications.
- After discharge, pay attention to the following:
- Rest and avoid heavy lifting or strenuous activities.
- Focus on carrying and breastfeeding the baby while resting in bed.

- Consider taking vitamins under medical supervision to replenish lost blood.
- Stay hydrated and consume nutritious meals rich in vitamins.
- Monitor the wound site and report any unusual changes to the doctor immediately.

Follow these restrictions after a Cesarean:

- Minimize stair-climbing.
- Avoid marital relations until consulting the doctor.
- Refrain from lifting anything heavier than the baby for the first two weeks.
- Avoid vaginal douches.
- Seek assistance for bending and standing tasks like laundry and cleaning.
- Avoid driving and frequent stair climbing.
- Consult a doctor before resuming exercise.

Balancing motherhood with other responsibilities

Do I have to take a bath after giving birth?
Yes, taking a warm bath immediately after giving birth is recommended, provided suitable facilities are available in the hospital. The bath should be taken in a warm environment to prevent catching a cold. If needed, a relative or nurse can assist you with this process.

How many sanitary pads should I have on hand after childbirth?

If you're giving birth in a hospital, the nurses will provide a disposable bed cover to protect against leaks. For home births, you'll need a protective cover for your bed to keep the mattress clean. Additionally, stock up on maternity pads as bleeding can be heavy initially. Change pads every 2 hours on the first day, then every 3-4 hours afterward. Purchase at least two or three packages containing 12 pads each for the time being.

Note:

- Go for maternity pads designed for postpartum use due to their absorbency and size.
- Don't forget to wash your hands before and after changing pads.

After the first few days, bleeding will decrease, changing from deep red to pink, then brown in the second and third weeks. Breastfeeding may temporarily increase bleeding due to uterine contractions. As bleeding lessens, regular pads can be used by the end of the first week, and panty liners may suffice by the fourth week.

When will monthly periods return after giving birth?

The return of menstruation after childbirth varies among women and is influenced by factors like breastfeeding. Breastfeeding mothers may experience delayed periods due to prolactin, a hormone that suppresses follicle-stimulating hormone (FSH) and luteinizing hormone (LH), which are responsible for ovulation.

This delay can last between six and twelve months, with menstrual pain possibly preceding the return of periods. The frequency of breastfeeding affects the duration of this delay.

Mothers who bottle-feed their babies typically resume menstruation one to three months after childbirth.

It's important to note that pregnancy can occur before menstruation resumes postpartum.

Marital relation after giving birth

Abstaining from marital relations for at least forty days, and possibly longer, is recommended to prevent infection in the womb.

Is it possible to take birth control pills while breastfeeding?

Using an alternative form of contraception is preferred because birth control pills can decrease milk production. During this period, breast milk is the sole source of nutrition for the baby.

Breastfeeding and your figure

Contrary to a common belief among many mothers, especially new ones, breastfeeding positively affects their appearance and figure.

It stimulates uterine contractions, reduces bleeding, and assists the uterus in returning to its normal size, consequently aiding in reducing the belly size. Additionally, breastfeeding facilitates the elimination of fat accumulated during pregnancy, restoring the woman's figure.

What's the most effective approach to postpartum weight loss?

Many mothers are eager to shed excess weight immediately after giving birth, but the postpartum period isn't the ideal time for weight loss, especially for breastfeeding mothers. Even if a lactating mother's diet is lacking in some aspects, it's unlikely to affect her milk production significantly.

However, inadequate nutrition may lead to a decrease in the mother's energy levels and could result in anemia. A nursing mother requires approximately 200 extra calories per day, on top of what she needs during pregnancy, to ensure an adequate milk supply for her baby and meet her nutritional requirements.

Maintaining your weight

While it's generally not advisable for a new mother to actively try to lose weight, there are measures she can take to maintain her weight and prevent weight gain. Here are some strategies:

Light exercise

Light exercises such as jogging and swimming can help strengthen abdominal and pelvic muscles. Aiming for 15 to 30 minutes of exercise at least three to five times a week is recommended.

If you didn't exercise during pregnancy, start with 15-minute sessions and gradually increase to 30 minutes. If you reduce exercise frequency during pregnancy, resume at the previous level and gradually increase. If you feel any discomfort, seek advice from your doctor.

Establishing eating habits that promote weight maintenance and ensure good health.

Dr. Judy Mazel emphasizes in her book, "Ideal Eating Habits, Better than Dieting," that weight gain isn't solely caused by increased food intake but rather by unhealthy eating habits. She suggests that certain food combinations are slowly absorbed, leading to fat accumulation, while others are quickly absorbed, providing energy and promoting a leaner body.

Maintaining an energetic and slender physique can enhance one's vitality and zest for life, as excess fat often leads to lethargy, which can be particularly challenging for women.

Eating breakfast, the most important meal of the day

Kickstart your day with breakfast; it aids weight loss by stimulating calorie burning. Go for options like iron and vitamin-fortified cornflakes. And remember to stay hydrated, aiming for at least 8 to 10 cups of water daily.

Starting your lunch with vegetable soup
Following breakfast, include plenty of salad in your meals, and after that, feel free to enjoy your favorite foods in moderation.
Not eating fats
It's best to avoid fats like vegetable oil, ghee, or butter and fried foods, not only due to their high-calorie content but also because they are unhealthy. While many women naturally lose weight through breastfeeding, this isn't the case for everyone, so don't expect rapid weight loss.
Consider the first year post-birth as a safe period to gradually return to your pre-pregnancy weight. Some famous women who appear to lose weight quickly may not prioritize their health or their children's.

Appropriate nutrition for a woman post childbirth

- Eat moderate portions.
- Include plenty of fresh and boiled fruits and vegetables to prevent hunger without consuming too many calories.
- Drink 8 to 12 cups of water daily, which is especially important for milk production during breastfeeding.
- Balance your meals by avoiding combining large amounts of proteins and carbohydrates in one sitting.
- opt for herbs, butter, or olive oil instead of ketchup and sauces.

- Indulge in your favorite foods in moderation to avoid feeling deprived and overeating later.
- Limit caffeine and avoid harmful substances like nicotine, which can pass into breast milk.
- Balance heavier meals with lighter options like yogurt and fruit the next day.
- Prioritize vegetables and fruits, but don't overdo it when pairing them with protein and carbohydrate-rich meals to prevent indigestion.
- Remove the skin from poultry before cooking to reduce fat intake.
- Skip dressings on salads and use less water when boiling vegetables to retain their nutritional value.
- Incorporate iron- and calcium-rich foods into your diet to support your body's needs during this period.

Postnatal exercises and the importance thereof

Exercise indeed offers numerous benefits for postpartum recovery:

- Exercise stimulates the release of endorphins, which can boost Mood and promote feelings of well-being.
- Regular exercise aids in shedding excess weight gained during pregnancy and helps in returning to pre-pregnancy weight.

- Physical activity can provide relief from discomfort by increasing energy levels and reducing feelings of fatigue.
- Exercise helps in building physical strength and endurance, which are essential for caring for a newborn and handling daily tasks.
- Research indicates that engaging in consistent physical activity could decrease the likelihood of postpartum depression by improving mental well-being and decreasing stress levels.

Types of exercise that are not recommended during the first few weeks after giving birth

- It's advisable to refrain from swimming until vaginal bleeding or discharge (lochia) has ceased, typically around seven days after giving birth.
- If you had a Cesarean section, it's essential to wait until your postpartum check-up, usually around six weeks after delivery, before starting any exercise regimen. Consult your doctor during this visit to determine suitable exercises for your recovery.

Advice to the new mother

It's important to avoid excessive exercise, particularly in the initial postpartum phase. While you might feel eager to work out intensely at first, it's vital to recognize the signs of postnatal depression or physical exhaustion. Starting with gentle exercise and taking breaks as needed is advisable. If you encounter any discomfort or urinary incontinence during physical activity, seeking guidance from your doctor is essential.

Exercises to strengthen the abdominal muscles
Pelvic exercises
Pelvic floor exercises
These workouts, known as Kegel exercises, prepare the pelvic floor muscles for childbirth and benefit you throughout your life. They involve contracting and releasing the pelvic floor muscles as if you're halting urination midway. Neglecting these muscles can result in weakened bladder control and urinary incontinence during activities like running, walking, laughing, or coughing.

Pelvic lift
This exercise is beneficial as it mobilizes and gently stretches the back while engaging the abdominal muscles, which can help alleviate back pain.

You can perform pelvic lift exercises while lying on your back, sitting, or using an exercise ball.

While lying on your back:

1. Lie on the ground or bed. Bend your knees and bring your feet close to your buttocks.
2. Contract the pelvic floor muscles and pull your lower abdominal muscles inward, then press your lower back into the floor or bed. Hold this position for a count of three, then lift your back off the surface. Repeat this exercise ten times, ensuring you breathe normally.

While sitting:

1. Sit on a straight-backed chair or a chair without a
    back, with your feet firmly on the ground.
2. Tighten your pelvic floor muscles and hold for a
    count of ten, then relax for a count of ten. Repeat
    this sequence ten times. Aim to do three sets of ten
    repetitions per day.

Using an exercise ball:

1. Sit on the exercise ball with your feet on the ground.
    It's advisable to place the ball on a mat to prevent
    slipping.
2. Move the ball forward and backward using your
    buttocks, allowing the pelvis to move while keeping
    your shoulders still. You can also move the ball
    from side to side to engage your waist muscles.

Your figure and girdles

Many women eager to regain their pre-pregnancy
figures often opt for shortcuts like girdles or corsets
without realizing the long-term consequences. While
these garments may benefit specific medical cases,
such as prolapsed kidneys or weakened abdominal
muscles post-surgery, they should only be prescribed
by a doctor and custom-made to fit the patient's body.

However, relying solely on girdles can weaken
abdominal muscles and lead to flabby skin. They
inhibit sweat evaporation, increasing the risk of skin

issues and fat accumulation due to reduced movement. Additionally, they can cause indigestion and constipation by compressing the abdomen and hindering intestinal activity. Poor circulation and vein pressure may also result, leading to visible veins.

Resorting to shortcuts may seem tempting, but it's crucial to prioritize long-term health and fitness over quick fixes.

Emotional care of the mother after giving birth

A mother's emotional and psychological well-being after giving birth is as crucial as her physical health. She may experience various emotions and challenges that could affect her psyche without adequate emotional support. Responsibilities increase significantly as she becomes solely responsible for caring for her newborn, alongside existing duties towards her husband and other children, and possibly work outside the home. Many women also struggle with body image concerns post-birth, feeling they've lost their previous beauty and figure.

These factors can profoundly impact a mother's mental health, necessitating adaptation to her new role to fulfill her duties effectively. The husband is vital in providing emotional support by understanding and alleviating her physical and psychological strain.

Creating a loving and supportive environment, assisting with childcare, and offering encouragement can significantly contribute to the mother's happiness and adjustment to this new phase of life.

Enjoy your child and overcome any feelings of distress or depression.

New mothers may experience feelings of distress and depression post-birth, influenced by various factors such as concerns about the baby's well-being, changes in appearance, and increased responsibilities. These emotions, known as postnatal depression, can be intensified by physiological changes in the body. It's important to recognize and address these feelings promptly, as they affect the mother, the baby, and the husband.

To combat these feelings, it's essential to remember the blessings of motherhood and seek enjoyment in spending time with the child. Sharing experiences with other mothers and engaging in joyful and fulfilling activities can help alleviate loneliness and boost morale. Open communication with the husband about loneliness and seeking childcare support can also be beneficial.

Furthermore, involvement in charitable activities and carving out personal time each day, regardless of circumstances, can contribute to overall well-being and self-care for the mother.

Going back to work

Many women express a desire to return to work soon after giving birth, often within three months or so, for various reasons:

1. **Career advancement:** Some women are eager to continue their career progression and fear missing out on opportunities if they take a prolonged break to care for their child. They worry that staying at home may slow down their career trajectory.
2. **Financial independence:** Others may want to maintain financial independence and not rely solely on their husband's income. They feel empowered by knowing they can support themselves financially if necessary.

However, deciding between prioritizing career aspirations and spending time with the new family can be challenging. Many women feel torn between these two priorities, especially as some employers may perceive a lack of commitment to work if they take extended leave for childcare responsibilities.

When is the right time to go back to work?

As the only one who can answer this question, it's important to consider several factors:

1. **Child's Health:** Consider your child's health first. Are there any health concerns or special needs that require your attention? If your child has health issues, you may need to prioritize their care and stay home longer.

2. **Support System:** Evaluate your support system. Do you have trusted family members, neighbors, or a reliable daycare facility that can care for your child in your absence? Having reliable childcare options can greatly influence your decision to return to work.

3. **Work Circumstances:** Assess your work circumstances. Is your job flexible enough to accommodate your needs as a new parent? Do you have the option to take a longer leave of absence if necessary, or is returning to work quickly a financial necessity?

4. **Personal Readiness:** Reflect on your readiness to balance work and home responsibilities. Are you mentally and emotionally prepared to juggle the demands of your job and caring for your child? Consider how returning to work will impact your overall well-being and family dynamics.

Considering all these factors, you can determine whether now is the right time for you to return to work or if it's best to delay your return until you feel more confident in your childcare arrangements and personal readiness.

Providing care for your newborn from birth to three months.

Now that you've become a mother to your newborn, a new phase of heightened responsibility begins toward your baby and your family. This responsibility demands innovative thinking and intelligence to raise your child into a successful, well-rounded individual. It's not an easy task.

This goal must take precedence over everything else in your life. Embrace your child with love and joy, dedicating ample time, effort, care, and affection, bringing you happiness and the warmth of maternal love in return. Therefore, you require some initial guidance on caring for your baby to help them develop into the unique individual you envision. Below, I'll provide advice and information to ensure your child's happiness.

Breastfeeding

The mother's breast milk is nature's perfect nourishment for infants, a divine gift placed by God within a woman's breasts. It provides the ideal blend of nutrients tailored to the infant's digestive system and growing body, offering a healthy start in life.

Breastfeeding supplies nourishment and fosters a loving bond between mother and child through touch, smell, and eye contact.

Despite advances in formula milk, it can never match the benefits of natural breast milk, as its nutrients are irreplaceable. The advantages of breastfeeding extend beyond physical health to emotional well-being.

Advantages of breastfeeding for both the mother and the baby

1. Breastfed children face lower risks of contagious diseases, as mother's milk contains antibodies against conditions like diarrhea and certain cancers.
2. Breastfeeding fosters a sense of comfort and psychological stability for the mother due to the strong bond with her child and the fulfillment of her maternal role.
3. Breastfeeding often delays the return of menstrual periods, contributing to birth spacing.
4. Breastfed children experience fewer urinary tract and ear infections compared to bottle-fed counterparts, who are at a fivefold higher risk.
5. Breastfeeding reduces the likelihood of childhood obesity compared to bottle feeding.
6. Breastfeeding may aid the mother in shedding excess pregnancy weight.
7. Breastfeeding nurtures a strong emotional attachment between mother and child through warmth, security, and love.

8. Mother's milk is stored safely and at the right temperature, away from contaminants, and delivered to the child in easily swallowed amounts.
9. Breastfeeding stimulates the uterus to contract back to its normal size and position, aiding postpartum recovery.
10. Breastfeeding decreases the risk of ovarian and breast cancer before menopause.
11. Breastfeeding reduces the likelihood of developing osteoporosis.
12. Breastfeeding lowers the risk of gestational diabetes and its progression to type II diabetes.
13. Breast milk, always available at the right temperature, is the sole nutritional requirement for infants in their early months.
14. Mother's milk is readily accessible, free, and requires no preparation or sterilization, saving time and effort.

The first feeding

We recommend that the new mother initiate breastfeeding as soon as possible after birth due to numerous benefits. One such advantage is the colostrum, the initial breast milk secretion rich in protein, vitamins, and minerals like potassium and sodium chloride, and lower fat content. Colostrum also contains antibodies not transferred during pregnancy and digestive enzymes suitable for the newborn's stomach in the early days.

Additionally, immediate breastfeeding aids uterine contraction, reducing the risk of postpartum hemorrhage.

Advice for the first days of breastfeeding

There's no need to fret over the small amounts of milk your breasts produce in the initial days after birth. Newborns don't require much fluid as they're born with water reserves. What's crucial for them are the proteins and antibodies found in the colostrum.

Does my baby need water?

Indeed, infants under six months old don't require water as they receive sufficient hydration from their mother's milk, which typically contains around 880 ml of water per liter, an ideal amount. Additionally, their immune systems aren't yet developed enough to combat potential contaminants in water, even minor ones.

Dr. Jennifer Anders, an emergency pediatric medicine specialist, highlights that excessive water intake in infants can lead to sodium loss, affecting brain function and potentially causing symptoms of water intoxication. However, in cases where significant water loss occurs due to factors like diarrhea, vomiting, or excessive sweating, it's crucial to restore hydration by addressing the underlying cause or supplementing with sterilized water between regular breastfeeding.

The correct position for breastfeeding

Ensuring your baby's correct positioning while breastfeeding is crucial to prevent nipple pain and facilitate milk flow.

It's recommended to have small pillows nearby before beginning breastfeeding, as they can provide support for your baby during the feeding process.

Latching on

- Bring your baby close to your breast; avoid bringing your breast close to your baby. Wait until the baby opens his mouth wide; if he only partially opens it, gently touch his upper lip with your nipple to encourage a wider opening.
- Ensure the baby takes the whole areola (the darker area around the nipple) into his mouth.
- You might need to place a finger on your breast to keep it slightly away from the baby's nose.

Signs that the baby has latched on to the nipple properly:

1. His lower lip is folded back beneath your nipple.
2. The baby's ears are moving while he is breastfeeding.
3. There is no pain in your nipple, or any pain felt is minimal.

If you feel your baby has not latched on properly, gently reposition him and offer the breast again correctly.

When you want to remove your nipple from the baby's mouth, you can gently insert your little finger into the corner of his mouth to break the suction.

How to breastfeed while lying down:

1. Lie down on your side with your baby facing you and his mouth in line with your breast.

2. Use pillows or cushions to support yourself and make yourself comfortable. Placing a pillow behind the baby's back can help keep him close to you.

This position gives you more control over the baby's head and is particularly helpful for women who have had a Caesarean section.

To know when your baby has had enough milk, watch for these signs:

1. Your breasts feel less heavy and softer after breastfeeding.
2. According to developmental standards, your baby's weight will gradually and naturally increase. Newborns typically lose approximately 10% of their birth weight during the first three days.
3. Your baby should have between six and eight wet diapers every twenty-four hours.
4. The baby's stools will be yellow in color.

Advice for increasing the milk supply

- Feed your baby whenever he shows signs of hunger, following a "feeding on demand" approach.
- Switch between breasts during each feeding session.
- Emptying your breasts using expression or pumping after breastfeeding can help stimulate more milk production by signaling the need for it to your body.
- Refrain from using contraceptive medications as they may diminish milk production. Consult your doctor for alternative contraceptive options suitable for breastfeeding.

- Stick to exclusively breastfeeding your baby without resorting to bottle milk supplementation. Your milk production will adjust according to your baby's feeding needs.

Expressing breast milk

Expressing milk involves removing milk from the breast using either hand expression or a breast pump machine. It's a useful method when direct breastfeeding isn't possible, allowing you to store milk later in bottles or cups in the fridge. Learning how to express milk is a skill that requires practice and can be beneficial for relieving swollen breasts and increasing milk supply.

If there are times when you can't breastfeed your baby, such as when taking medication that might affect your baby or during a hospital stay, expressing milk helps maintain milk production levels. This prevents a decrease in milk supply if you stop breastfeeding abruptly without expressing milk, ensuring an adequate supply when you resume breastfeeding and avoiding the need for supplementary bottle feeding.

Reasons for expressing breast milk:

1. If the baby is in the neonatal intensive care unit, such as due to premature birth or illness.
2. When nipple issues prevent direct breastfeeding, such as cracked or inverted nipples or nipple pain.
3. To alleviate breast swelling.

4. If returning to work and unable to bring the baby along.
5. When away from home for extended periods, like visiting relatives or traveling, and leaving the baby with a caregiver.
6. To sustain milk production levels during a breastfeeding hiatus due to illness.

In any circumstance, expressing breast milk is the most suitable alternative to direct breastfeeding when needed.

How to express milk from the breast:

The mother can express milk using her hand or specialized machines designed for this purpose. Regardless of the method chosen, it's considered a skill that requires some training and practice, improving with experience over time.

Expressing milk by hand

This cost-effective method doesn't require any special equipment and can save time. Many women prefer this approach and quickly become accustomed to it.

Here's how to do it:

1. Wash your hands thoroughly with soap and water.
2. Use a sterilized vessel to collect the milk.
3. Position your fingers around the nipple, about 2.5-3.5 centimeters away, forming a C-shape with your fingers and thumb around the areola.
4. Gently squeeze your fingers and thumb together while moving your hand backward toward the chest wall.

5. Follow this with a circular movement around the areola.

Note: Avoid placing your thumb and fingers too close to the nipple to prevent pain during squeezing.

Vacuum pumps

There are two types of breast pumps:

1. **Manual pumps:** These are operated by squeezing a lever or plunger.

2. **Mechanical pumps:** These are powered by batteries or mains electricity and are quicker and more effective.

To use a breast pump:

- Place the suction cup over the breast before turning the pump on, allowing it to express and pump the milk into the connected container.

Notes:

- Ensure the nipple is in the middle of the disk or cup over the breast.
- It should move in and out with each pump without causing pain.
- Ensure the whole breast moves and the nipple isn't rubbing against the cup inside.
- Using a two-headed pump is preferable as it's quicker, easier, and can increase milk production.
- If using a single pump, switch it from one breast to the other several times.
- Keep expressing as long as milk flows to ensure your baby receives the fatty milk.

Storing expressed breast milk

You can store expressed milk in sterilized plastic containers designed for this purpose or in plastic bags. Freshly pumped breast milk stored in the refrigerator should be used within twenty-four hours. Frozen milk should be used for no longer than three months.

To defrost frozen milk, place the bottle or bag in a vessel of warm water and run warm water from the tap over it. You can also defrost it in the refrigerator overnight. It is better not to use the microwave or bottle warmer because these two methods can reduce the nutrients in the mother's milk.

Contradictions for breastfeeding

Breastfeeding plays a crucial role in the growth and development of the baby, and it also holds significance for the mother's well-being, as discussed earlier. However, there are instances where breastfeeding may not be suitable, with reasons about the mother, the baby, or both. The most notable reasons include:

Factors that may prevent the mother from breastfeeding:

- If the mother has a disease that could potentially affect the baby, such as tuberculosis, which can be transmitted through touch or the respiratory system.
- Chronic diseases that drain the mother's strength, like heart disease, cancer, kidney disease, liver disease, and anemia, may hinder breastfeeding.
- Contagious diseases like typhoid or lung infections can also prevent breastfeeding.

- If the mother becomes pregnant again, it's preferred for her to stop breastfeeding after the fifth month to avoid physiological strain.
- It's advisable to address inverted nipples before breastfeeding.
- In cases of nipple damage, breastfeeding should be paused for 2 to 4 days, or a nipple shield may be used after consulting a doctor.

Factors preventing the baby from breastfeeding:

- Ulcers in the baby's mouth.
- Heart or lung disease.
- Neurological problems that result in a weak sucking reflex.
- Prematurely born children may not have developed the ability to suck effectively.

Bottle Feeding

This type of feeding is termed "feeding out of necessity," I only recommend it in cases of urgent need, such as when circumstances prevent breastfeeding, as mentioned previously.

Note: If you desire to breastfeed your baby but find your breast milk insufficient, it's important to continue breastfeeding while consulting a doctor regarding the use of bottled milk as a supplement. In such cases, bottle feeding can be pursued, and both parents can participate.

Types of baby formula (artificial milk)
Ready-made milk

is available in disposable bottles, offering the convenience of no mixing required. It comes in sterile containers, eliminating the need to add potentially contaminated water, which is particularly beneficial in developing countries. However, it's costly and must be used within 48 hours of opening.

Liquid concentrate milk

requires careful adherence to instructions, as an incorrect ratio of milk to water can strain the infant's kidneys or affect their nutrition and growth.

Dried or powdered formula

sold in cans with measuring spoons, is less expensive, and doesn't need refrigeration once opened. However, it must be consumed within a month after opening, and the mother must try to mix it with water thoroughly. Following instructions precisely and accurately measuring the amounts of water and formula is essential.

Equipment needed for bottle feeding

1. Bottles: Purchase ten 250 ml bottles to accommodate the feeding needs.
2. Teats: Acquire a variety of teats, available in different types such as traditional, orthodontic (designed to minimize pressure on developing teeth and gums), and flat-topped (emulating the shape of the breast).

3. Measuring jug: Utilize a measuring jug to accurately measure the amount of water required based on the quantity of powder or concentrated milk to be added to the bottle.

4. Plastic funnel: Use a plastic funnel to pour the prepared milk into the bottle without spillage.

5. Plastic spoon: Keep a plastic spoon handy for mixing the milk thoroughly in the bottle before feeding.

A few words of advice

- Avoid heating bottles in the microwave to prevent the risk of the bottle or teat becoming too hot and potentially burning the child's mouth.

- Don't leave leftover milk in the bottle for an extended period without washing it. It's advisable to empty any remaining milk and soak the bottle in water until you can wash it properly.

- If milk remains after feeding, discard it or refrigerate it immediately after the baby has finished feeding.

- Take all necessary precautions to thoroughly clean and sterilize bottles to prevent contamination that could harm your baby's health.

Sterilizing bottles

To properly sterilize equipment for bottle feeding and ensure no germs enter the baby's system, the following steps are recommended:

1. Use sterilizing liquid or tablets available at pharmacies and add them to cold water in a sterilization container.
2. Utilize a dedicated bottle brush to clean the bottles from the inside. This brush should be solely used for this purpose, not other cleaning tasks.
3. Clean the inside of the teats using table salt.
4. Have a container designated for sterilization, where the cold water and sterilizing liquid are combined.

Sterilizing bottles: tried, tested, and proper method

1. Wash the bottles and teats in hot water, using a brush designed for cleaning bottles to remove all traces of milk.
2. Scrub the inside of the teats with salt to eliminate any remaining milk residue.
3. Rinse all equipment in cold water, including bottles and teats.
4. Use a pin to clean the hole in the teat.
5. Prepare a sterilization bucket with cold water and add sterilizing liquid or tablets. Place the equipment into the bucket.
6. Stir the equipment in the sterilization solution, then seal the bucket with its lid.
7. Allow the equipment to soak in the sterilized water for some time; remove items as needed and let them air dry.

Other methods of sterilizing bottles

Many electrical appliances are available in the market and are designed specifically for sterilizing bottles, teats, and other feeding equipment using steam, microwave technology, and other methods. These appliances offer convenience and efficiency, potentially saving time and effort compared to traditional sterilization methods.

Preparing bottles

1. Boil water.
2. Measure and pour the appropriate amount of hot water into the bottle according to the instructions on the formula container.
3. Add the correct amount of formula powder to the water in the bottle using the provided scoop.
4. Secure the lid on the bottle and shake vigorously until the powder is completely dissolved.
5. Attach the teat to the bottle without touching the part in the baby's mouth, then allow it to cool to the appropriate temperature.
6. Ensure the bottle is at body temperature (35-37°C) before offering it to the baby.

Note:

If a new teat restricts the milk flow and is too slow for your baby, widen the hole using a sterilized pin or needle. If this doesn't resolve the issue, you can create additional holes.

Avoid forcing your baby to feed beyond feeling full, as his appetite may vary from one meal to another. Forcing him to eat more may have the opposite effect and lead to loss of appetite.

Burping

Your baby will naturally swallow some air while feeding, so it's important to burp him to help release this air, preventing potential indigestion or the feeling of fullness when he hasn't had enough to eat. Here are several ways to burp your baby:

1. Place him gently face down on your lap.
2. Lift him until his chest rests on your shoulder, then gently rub or pat his back.
3. Hold your baby upright with his head slightly tilted forward while supporting his neck and back, then gently pat his back as shown in the picture.
4. He may spit up some of the milk, so putting a bib on him and placing a receiving blanket or small, soft towel on your lap or shoulder to keep clothes clean and make cleanup easier.

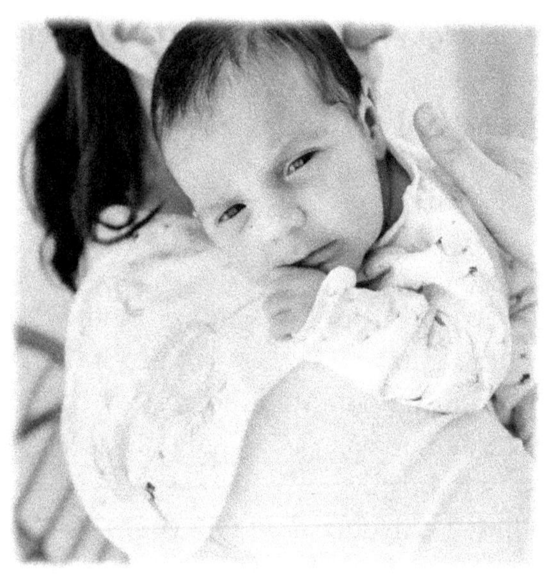

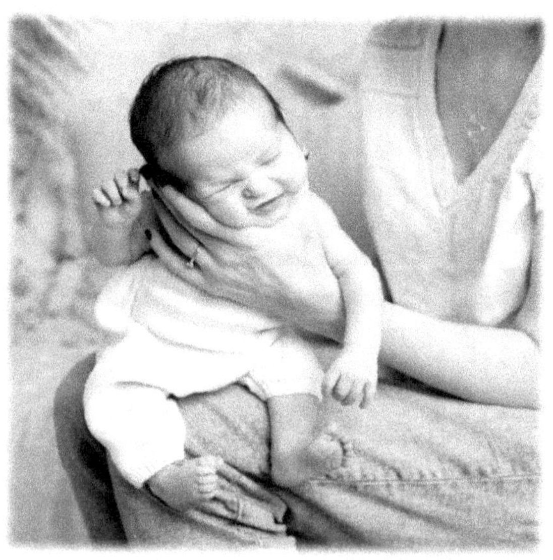

Bathing

Before beginning to bathe your baby, ensure you have everything you need to be prepared:

1. A tub of warm water.
2. Mild soap and shampoo designed for infants, ensuring they are safe for their delicate skin.
3. A soft sponge or flannel to gently wash your baby's skin.
4. A soft towel to wrap your baby in after the bath.
5. Clean diaper and clothes to dress your baby after bathing.

Once you have everything ready, you can proceed with bathing your baby.

step-by-step guide to bathing your baby

1. Remove your baby's clothes from the top half and clean his nose, ears, eyes, and face using a soft sponge or flannel suitable for infants.
2. Remove the clothes from your baby's lower half and clean his stomach and genitals as usual.
3. Lower the baby gently into the water and start bathing him.
4. Wash the baby's head with water and mild shampoo or soap, avoiding perfumed products.
5. Wash the baby's body with water and mild soap, carefully cleaning folds and creases.

6. Rinse the baby's body and lift him safely onto a soft towel to gently dry him.

7. If the umbilical cord or circumcision has not healed, give your baby a sponge bath instead, ensuring clean folds on the skin in the neck area.

8. Avoid pulling on the baby's umbilical cord before it falls off naturally to prevent bleeding.

9. Bathe and dress the baby in the same room to avoid exposing him to drafts.

10. Schedule the bath half an hour before breastfeeding.

11. Keep the bath short, not exceeding five minutes, to prevent the baby from catching a cold.

12. Interact with your baby and talk to him during his bath to leave him with a positive impression of bathing and water.

13. Apply cream on your baby's bottom to prevent diaper rash, followed by suitable oil all over his body to moisturize it.

14. Avoid using cologne or perfumed substances to prevent skin infections.

15. Ensure the water temperature is between 36°C and 37°C, and never leave the baby unattended in the water. Avoid adding hot water to the tub while the baby is in it.

Cleaning the parts of your baby's body (sponge bath)

A sponge bath is another method of cleaning your baby, where you clean each body part separately. This approach is suitable for situations where the child is sick, has low weight, or feels very nervous in water. It allows for gentle cleaning without the need for immersion in water.

Below are some ways of cleaning your baby's body bit by bit

Skin

It's common for various spots and rashes to appear on your newborn's skin, most of which will naturally disappear over time.
However, if a skin rash persists, it could indicate a medical issue, and it's important to consult a doctor.

Use a soft sponge or flannel dampened with lukewarm water to clean your baby's skin. Gently rub the baby's skin with the sponge, then pat it dry with a soft towel. Finally, apply a children's oil suitable for moisturizing the skin. This routine helps maintain your baby's skin health and cleanliness.

Eyes

To clean each eye separately, dampen a piece of cotton wool with warm (not hot) water for each eye. Gently wipe from the inside corner to the outside edge of the eye. This helps remove debris or discharge while ensuring hygiene and comfort for your baby.

Ears

When cleaning your baby's ears, focus on the outside and inside of the ear, avoiding the ear canal. Use a soft cloth or flannel to avoid cotton buds or Q-Tips™, which could potentially damage the delicate eardrum.

Nose

To clean your baby's nose, use a cloth or flannel to wipe gently around each nostril from the outside. This helps maintain cleanliness and hygiene without risking injury to the delicate nasal passages.

Nails

Clipping your baby's nails while they're asleep can be easier, helping to prevent accidental scratches. It's important to make this a regular part of your routine to ensure your baby's nails stay trimmed and prevent any accidental scratching.

Navel (bellybutton)

Once the umbilical cord falls off, the area may appear incompletely healed and could take several days or weeks to fully heal. No dressing is necessary for this unhealed area, but keeping it clean and dry is crucial to prevent infection. Keeping it dry aids in skin formation until it fully heals. After the cord stump falls off, your baby can safely take baths in the tub. When changing diapers, fold the top edge to expose the umbilical area and keep it dry until it heals. If you notice any discharge or redness around the area, it's essential to consult a doctor for further evaluation.

Diapers (nappies)

There's a wide variety of diaper options available, allowing mothers to choose what works best for them and their baby's needs. Some mothers prefer using cloth diapers at home for sustainability reasons while opting for disposable diapers when traveling or outside with the baby for convenience.

It's all about finding the right balance and what works best for the baby and the parent's lifestyle.

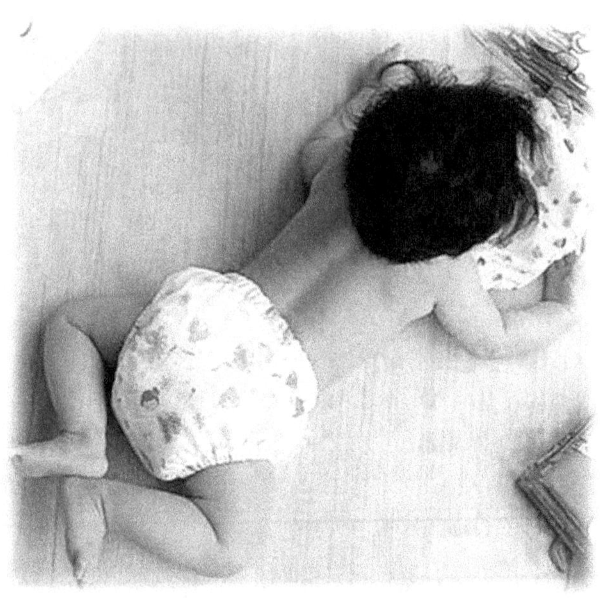

Types of diapers

Disposable diapers

Disposable diapers are indeed preferred by many mothers for their convenience and ease of use.

With various sizes available to suit the baby's growth stages, they provide a hassle-free solution for diaper changing.

Cloth diapers

Cloth diapers offer a reusable and environmentally friendly option for diapering.

There's a wide range of options, from traditional flat diapers to modern fitted designs in various colors and patterns. Some mothers also opt for disposable liners to enhance convenience and cleanliness.

Changing diaper 1

- Regular diaper changes are crucial to maintaining cleanliness and preventing diaper rash, especially after bowel movements.
- After cleaning, applying a protective cream like Vaseline can help prevent irritation. Avoid perfumed wipes or cortisone creams, and don't fasten the diaper too tightly to allow ventilation.
- Let the baby go without a diaper whenever possible to promote airflow and reduce the risk of infection.

Things you will need when changing a diaper

1. Cloths or flannels for cleaning.
2. A jug of warm water with a small amount of mild soap for washing.
3. Barrier cream to protect the baby's skin.
4. Water-resistant cream like zinc cream with castor oil to prevent moisture.
5. Non-perfumed wet wipes designed for infants for on-the-go cleaning. Avoid applying talcum powder over cream-applied areas.

Changing the diaper 2

- Gather all necessary supplies before starting.
- Never leave the baby unattended on a changing table or bed.
- Lift the baby's back by holding onto his ankles to prevent movement.
- Roll up the dirty diaper halfway under the baby.
- Lift the baby's legs and carefully clean his bottom.
- Use a damp cloth or wet wipe to clean your child from front to back, reducing the risk of infection, especially for girls.
- Lift your baby's legs and clean his behind.
- Lay your baby on his back and lift him slightly to place half the new diaper beneath him.
- Bring the other half between his legs and fold the upper part beneath his belly button if it's not yet healed properly.
- Fasten the diaper securely to avoid leaks.
- Wash your hands thoroughly after changing the diaper.

Protecting the baby from diaper rash

To prevent diaper area infections and protect your baby's skin, follow these steps:

1. Change the diaper promptly each time the baby urinates to keep the skin dry.
2. Allow some diaper-free time for your baby each day to let air reach the skin.

3. Avoid fastening the diaper too tightly to allow airflow.
4. Apply a protective cream, such as zinc oxide, to the skin to prevent dampness and irritation.
6. If the skin rash persists for an extended period, consult a doctor for further evaluation and treatment.

Dressing your baby

When purchasing clothes for your baby, consider the following:

- Ensure the clothes keep the baby comfortably warm without causing overheating or sweating, which can lead to dehydration.
- Avoid buying too many clothes as babies grow quickly; opt for practical options over fancy ones.
- Choose easy-to-fasten pants made of soft, flexible material and machine washable.
- Cotton clothes are preferred for easy cleaning, softness, and breathability.
- Avoid clothes with drawstrings and large collars to prevent the risk of strangulation.
- go for loose-fitting clothes to allow for proper ventilation and prevent the deformation of growing bones.

Tips and tricks for dressing your baby

- Ensure you have all the necessary clothing items and accessories within reach before you start.

- Choose a time when the baby is calm and not crying, preferably after feeding and napping.
- Distract the baby by playing with them or hanging toys or a mobile nearby to keep them engaged.
- Lay the baby down on a comfortable surface like a bed or changing table to make dressing easier and more comfortable for them.

Dressing the baby step-by-step

1. Open the neck of the vest as much as possible and pass the back under the baby's head. Bring the front down to his neck, then lift his head and pull the back of the vest downwards until it is level with his shoulders.
2. Put your hand in one of the sleeves and pull the child's arm through it. Repeat the same with the other arm.
3. Pull the front of the garment down to the baby's stomach, lift his legs, and pull the lower part of the vest down. Finally, fasten the two ends of the vest together.

Carrying your baby

The mother must handle her baby safely, especially in the early days when the baby's head and limbs are delicate. When picking up the baby, support his head by placing one hand under his neck and the other beneath his bottom. If lifting from the ground, kneel first, then follow the same steps. Avoid lifting the child by his arms or sides.

When standing or walking, cradle the baby's head in the crook of your elbow, keeping it slightly higher than the rest of his body, with your other arm wrapped around his back.

Alternatively, carry the baby with his upper half against your chest and his chest against your shoulder, supporting his head with one hand and his back with the other.

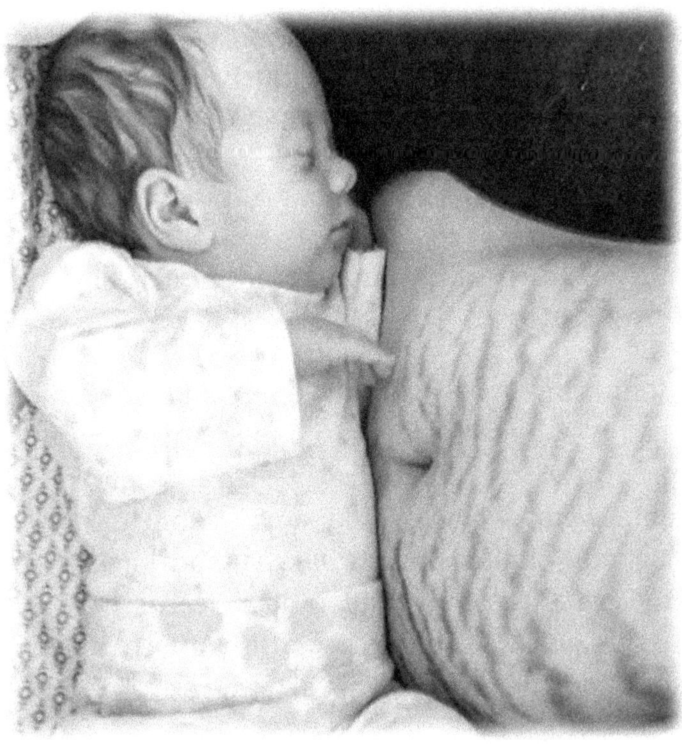

High temperature

High temperature, or fever, is the body's defense against sickness. When the body detects foreign invaders like bacteria or viruses, white blood cells, known as defensive cells, engage in battle to destroy them. In intense battles, the defensive cells signal the brain to raise body temperature, which can kill certain bacteria. Fever also prompts the body to produce more white blood cells to aid in the fight against invaders. Therefore, high temperature is both a response to illness and a sign of a problem or sickness in the body.

When should I be worried about my baby's temperature?

Monitoring a baby's body temperature is crucial. A healthy baby typically has a temperature between 36.5 and 37.7°C. Infants may have slightly higher temperatures than toddlers, and temperatures often fluctuate, higher during the day and lower at night. However, if a baby's temperature exceeds 37.8°C and is accompanied by distress or discomfort, it warrants attention and may indicate an issue.

Common causes for a baby's high temperature

High temperature in children typically signals an infection, with the specific illness varying. Here are common scenarios where a child might experience high temperature:

- Fever following vaccination
- Contracting colds or flu
- Developing throat or ear infections
- Upper respiratory tract infections or bronchitis
- Viral infections
- Urinary tract infections

Treating high temperature in the infant

1. Dress your infant in lightweight cotton garments.
2. For infants older than two months, administer the appropriate medication prescribed by a doctor to lower their temperature.
3. Ensure proper ventilation in the room and consider using air conditioning or a fan to create a cooler environment.
4. Place your baby in a lukewarm water bath and avoid drying them afterward.
5. Monitor your baby's diet and offer ample liquids.

Heat Rash

Heat rash manifests as red pimples or spots on the child's skin, typically around the neck, under the armpits, on the chest, in the diaper area, or under tight clothing. It may also occur on the child's forehead, indicating high body temperature. Heavy clothing or high ambient temperatures often contribute to this condition.

In hot and humid weather, children tend to sweat more profusely. Excessive sweating can result in sweat not properly evaporating through the skin pores due to their small size and the tightness of clothing. Consequently, trapped sweat forms a heat rash characterized by red spots on the skin.

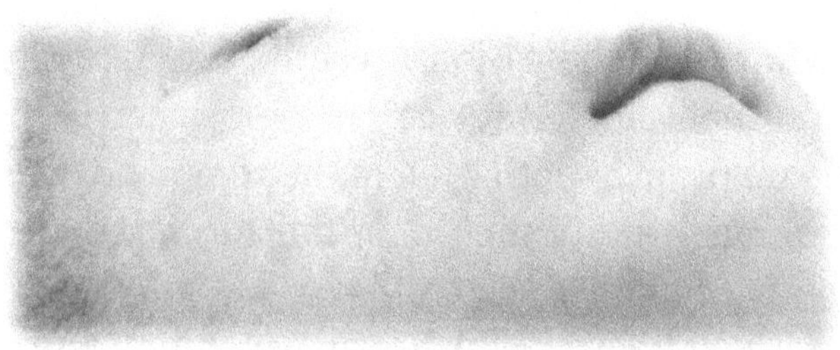

Protection against heat Rash

- When it's hot, use light, breathable clothing to prevent excessive sweating.
- Avoid taking your child outdoors in hot weather.

- Ensure proper ventilation and cooling in your child's bedroom using a fan or air conditioning during hot weather.
- Dermatologists recommend natural fabrics like cotton over synthetic ones for better sweat absorption.

How can I treat my child if he has a heat rash?

1. Remove some of the child's clothing to help them feel cooler, and consider letting them go naked occasionally.
2. Cool the affected area by applying cold cloths or placing the child in a lukewarm water tub, which can help alleviate heat rash.
3. Apply calamine lotion or hydrocortisone cream to the affected area to soothe irritation.
4. If the rash spreads or does not improve within 3 to 4 days, seek advice from a doctor.

Understanding newborn cries and soothing techniques

Crying

Crying is the primary way your child communicates his needs and desires, as it's his only form of expression. Generally, babies cry because they require something specific from you. Initially, crying may lack tears and be less expressive, but over the first few months, it develops into various tones that convey different messages.

As time passes, mothers become adept at distinguishing their baby's cries based on experience, allowing them to identify their baby's needs from the tone of their crying. Below is a more thorough discussion of this.

How much do babies cry on average?

Based on research by the Thomas Coram Research Unit at the University of London, a healthy baby typically cries for about two hours a day during the first three months of life. If crying exceeds three hours daily, it's considered excessive, and consulting a doctor is advisable.

Hunger

When your baby cries, hunger is often the primary reason. If you suspect hunger, promptly offer milk. Insufficient milk production from your breasts or inadequate feeding from a bottle could be caused. When breastfeeding, allow your baby to nurse until satisfied. If bottle-feeding, offer milk or diluted fruit juice.

Pain

Babies cry when they experience pain, contrary to the misconception that their nervous system is underdeveloped and they don't feel pain. Modern studies have shown that babies indeed feel pain, even in the womb, as their nervous system is fully developed. You can observe signs of pain in your baby through their movements. When in pain, babies may wave their arms and legs, and if the pain intensifies, they may draw their knees up to their tummy.

Temperature

It's essential to monitor your baby constantly to ensure they're neither too hot nor too cold. While the arms and legs may not accurately indicate your baby's temperature, placing your hand on their tummy is the best way to assess it. If you feel their temperature is elevated, it's important to consult a doctor promptly. Conversely, if your baby feels cold, this can also lead to crying. Dress your baby appropriately for the temperature, whether hot or cold.

Wet diaper

It is crucial to recognize when your baby needs a diaper change, as wetness can greatly bother them. Ensure the diaper pins are properly fastened to prevent any discomfort or leaks.

Sudden changes

Sudden changes in your baby's environment, like loud noises or bright lights, can cause distress or anxiety, leading to crying.

Feeling lonely

Your baby may cry when feeling bored from being left alone for extended periods without interaction or company. Avoid leaving your baby alone for too long to prevent boredom.

Fear of strangers

For your baby, a stranger is anyone they aren't accustomed to seeing regularly, even if it's their father. This is a natural response in infants.

Dealing with colic and sleep disturbances

Colic

Colic is often cited as one of the primary causes of crying in infants up to three months old. It's not an illness; typically, there's no underlying medical issue. However, consulting a doctor can offer reassurance and rule out any potential medical concerns. During a colic episode, the baby may pull their knees towards their stomach, turn red in the face, and cry continuously despite efforts to soothe them. They may briefly calm down, only to resume crying shortly after.

Causes that may lead to colic

- Imbalance in milk quantity or temperature, whether too much or too little or if the milk is too hot or cold, particularly in bottle-fed babies.
- Gas buildup in the intestines due to certain milk ingredients that the baby's body struggles to digest. Additionally, some foods consumed by the mother, like onions and garlic, can lead to gas in breastfed babies as these substances pass into the breast milk.
- Sensitivity of the baby's nervous system during the initial three months after birth.

- Psychological issues experienced by the mother during pregnancy.

How to deal with colic

- Ensure you consult a doctor to rule out any underlying sickness causing the colic.
- Gently massage the baby's tummy to alleviate discomfort.
- Offer the baby affection and physical contact. Hugging, patting, and engaging in affectionate activities can soothe the baby and provide a distraction from colic. Even if the crying persists, continue comforting and touching the baby.
- Recognize and accept your child's temperament. Some babies may be more prone to distress and may cry frequently for various reasons or no apparent reason due to their immature nervous and digestive systems. Stay patient, avoid getting frustrated, and provide consistent affection and support, hoping the situation will improve over time.

A few words of advice

1. Check your baby's diaper to see if it needs changing.
2. Ensure your baby is not hungry or thirsty.
3. Make sure your baby is comfortable regarding temperature.
4. Check for signs of illness in your baby.

5. Gently rock your baby in your arms or a swinging cradle.
6. Take your baby for a walk outside.
7. Provide entertainment, such as turning on the radio or TV when your baby is bored.
8. Shower your baby with love and affection.
9. Allow the baby's father to care for the baby occasionally to give yourself a break. Consider having separate sleeping arrangements so that the parents and baby can take turns resting.
10. Accept that crying is a natural part of infancy and serves to communicate your baby's needs.

Determine your baby's problem from the sound of his crying

To determine your baby's needs based on their crying, observe the following cues:

- Hunger: Short cries with consistent rising and falling of volume.
- Anger: The cry expresses upset and appears angry.
- Distress: Varied cry patterns, alternating between loud and long with pauses, then persistent crying with a level tone.
- Colic: Loud cries that may persist for hours.

Trust your intuition and respond accordingly to your baby's cues.

God has endowed mothers with warm compassion towards their children and a strong inclination to hold them gently and revel in their love. A baby needs these essential elements in their first year of life.

Some scientific studies once suggested that mothers should limit carrying their children excessively to avoid them becoming accustomed to it. They also recommended enforcing regular sleep schedules and letting babies cry without intervention to prevent dependency on being held. However, these approaches led to increased aggression, emotional issues, and temperament problems in children.

Nowadays, scientific research advocates responding promptly to a baby's cries, comforting them with affection and reassurance, and breastfeeding whenever needed, day or night. Addressing these psychological needs is crucial for a child's emotional well-being and development. Love, compassion, and attentive care ensure a child's healthy emotional growth and stability.

Say no to emotional weaning.

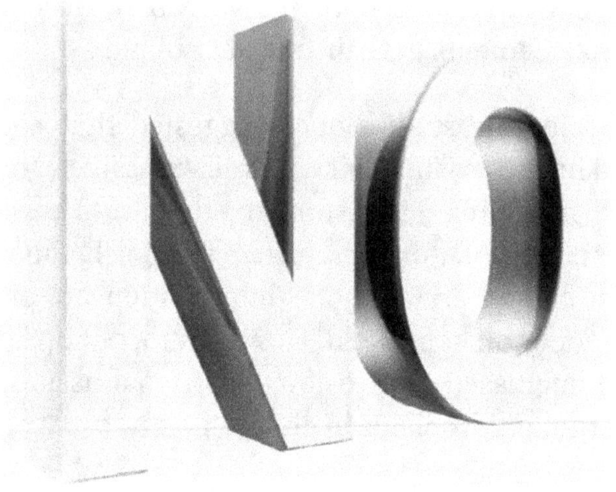

If a mother weans her baby from breastfeeding too soon, she deprives them of the natural nutrition provided by God. Similarly, withholding emotional and social care deprives the child of their natural right to compassion. Emotional weaning is considered more serious than early physical weaning.

Ignore anyone suggesting you spoil your baby by offering affection and care. Instead, embrace your child, shower them with kisses, tickle their feet, and always keep them close to you. These acts nurture emotional bonds and are essential for your baby's well-being.

From the earliest months, babies can perceive whether they are loved and welcomed by the family based on the care, love, and compassion shown towards them. Neglect and indifference will make the baby feel ignored and unloved.

These early experiences profoundly shape the baby's psychology and feelings and contribute to their strength of character and self-confidence. Your role is to remain patient and calm and attend to your baby's basic needs: breastfeeding, changing diapers, bathing, and playing with them.

Despite the challenges, you'll soon find yourself cherishing this stage, perhaps even desiring to have more children. It's all part of the nature with which God has endowed you.

A few words of advice

1. Keep the communication flowing with your baby; talking to them and engaging in physical contact is crucial for strengthening your bond.
2. Enhance communication by making eye contact and getting close to your baby during feeding or playtime.
3. Prioritize closeness with your husband to ensure he doesn't feel neglected. Many fathers may perceive a loss of interest when their wives are preoccupied

with the newborn. Allocate dedicated time daily for
both your baby and your husband.

4. Encourage your husband to actively participate in
    caring for the baby.

Sleep

Your baby's sleep needs are essential, and you can't
force them to sleep more or less than their body
requires. Understanding their sleep patterns is key,
allowing you to adapt your schedule to theirs and
ensuring you both get adequate rest. Creating a
tranquil environment free from noise disturbances is
crucial for their peaceful sleep.

Avoid running the washing machine or vacuum cleaner
near their sleeping area, as these noises disrupt their
rest.

Average sleep time of babies

Your baby's sleep duration varies; only they can
determine how long they sleep. Newborns typically
sleep between sixteen and twenty hours daily, waking
up every 3 or 4 hours due to hunger. During the first
two months, your baby's sleep pattern may seem
random, with more sleep during the day and waking
frequently at night. This is normal as they are too
young to distinguish between night and day. Over time,

they will gradually develop a more consistent sleep pattern.

Is it preferable for the mother to sleep next to her child?

When deciding where your baby should sleep, you should consider your own sleeping habits and any medications you take that might affect your sleep. If you typically sleep deeply or are on medication that influences your sleep, having your baby sleep in a crib nearby is advisable. This precaution minimizes the risk of accidentally rolling over onto your baby at night, although such incidents are rare among mothers. On the other hand, if you're a light sleeper who doesn't move around much during the night, there's no compelling reason why your baby shouldn't sleep beside you during the initial three months of life.

Where should the newborn baby sleep?

Newborns benefit from sleeping near their parents but shouldn't share the same bed. The ideal sleeping arrangement for a baby is to have a bassinet or crib placed close to the parent's bed.

Bassinet

The bassinet offers several advantages, including its practicality and portability, allowing it to easily move from one room to another. It should also provide a comfortable sleeping space for the baby, and adding an attractive lining can enhance its appeal.

Crib

Once your baby outgrows the bassinet or becomes more active and moves around a lot, it's time to transition him to the crib. While some parents choose to use the crib right from the beginning instead of a bassinet, it's important to note that, unlike the bassinet, the crib isn't portable and cannot be easily moved from one room to another.

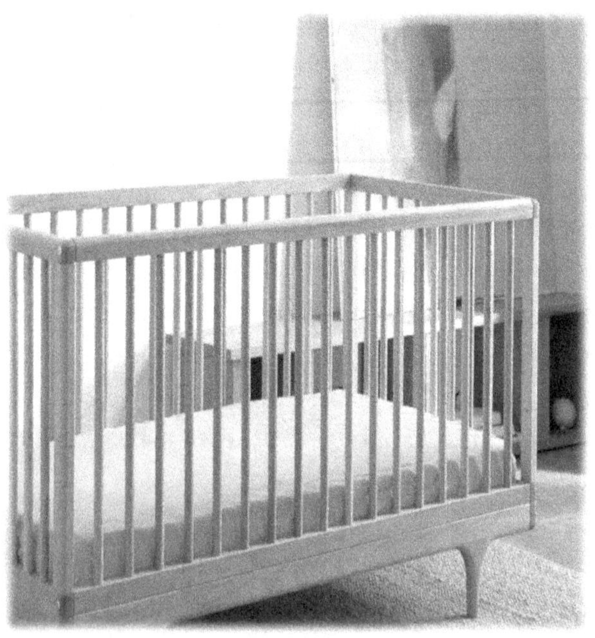

Safety concerns

To ensure the crib's safety and functionality, it's important to consider the following aspects:

1. The crib should be well-built and durable to withstand long-term use, especially if you use it for subsequent children.
2. Opting for a crib that allows rocking or swinging can comfort the baby. However, ensuring the crib is stable and won't tip over when in motion. Additionally, it should have the option to be immobilized when the baby is sleeping to prevent any accidents.
3. The crib should come with a firm, flat mattress that fits snugly into the crib. This ensures a safe sleeping surface for the baby and reduces the risk of suffocation or entrapment hazards.

How to keep the baby safe when he is sleeping

1. Avoid heavy blankets or soft mattresses, as they can cause the baby to become too hot. go for thin, cellular blankets and securely tuck the ends under the mattress to prevent suffocation.
2. Always keep the baby's head uncovered while sleeping to maintain airflow.
3. Position the baby with their feet touching the foot of the crib to prevent slipping beneath the blanket

and to keep their head safe from hitting the crib's end when picked up.

4. Regularly clean and air out the baby's mattress to maintain hygiene, ensuring it remains dry. To prevent entrapment hazards, check for gaps between the mattress and the crib's edge.
5. Remove toys or other items from the crib to reduce the risk of suffocation or choking hazards.

Should the baby sleep on his back or on his tummy?

Recent studies have indicated that placing babies to sleep on their backs reduces the risk of sudden infant death syndrome (SIDS) while sleeping on their tummies increases this risk due to the potential for suffocation when the baby's mouth is close to the mattress. Most babies naturally prefer sleeping on their backs, which is also considered safe for healthy infants. Sleeping on their sides poses a higher risk as babies may roll over onto their tummies during sleep. Therefore, it is crucial to encourage your baby to sleep on their back from the outset to promote safety and reduce the risk of SIDS.

Do babies dream?

Scientists have yet to determine whether babies dream, although it is widely speculated that they do indeed dream.

Is it advisable to allow my baby to cry alone until he falls asleep?

Babies often cry when left alone before sleeping, out of fear, or as a protest against being left unattended. Their crying serves as a means of attracting their mother's attention and expressing their unspoken needs and emotions. Ignoring a baby's cries can make them feel unsafe and alone, which can gradually affect their psychological well-being and contradict a mother's innate compassion. Therefore, it's advisable for mothers not to leave their baby crying alone for extended periods or until they fall asleep, as it can significantly impact the baby's psychology. However, if the baby wakes up crying, allowing them to cry briefly before comforting them with gentle gestures, such as patting them and showing compassion, is acceptable.

How will I know when my baby feels sleepy and that he is ready to go to sleep?

There are several signals indicating whether your baby is ready to sleep:

1. Slowing down of movements.
2. Staring at something in front of them even when there's nothing there.
3. Yawning.
4. Rubbing their eyes.
5. Losing interest in people around them and their toys.
6. Becoming irritable.
7. Leaning their head into your chest.

Types of sleep and waking in newborns

Deep, peaceful sleep
This stage is called non-rapid eye movement (NREM) sleep. It comprises four steps: drowsiness, light sleep, deep sleep, and very deep sleep, all of which happen gradually. During the deep sleep stage, there is minimal outward movement, and it's when the sleep hormone is produced.

Active sleep
This phase is termed rapid eye movement sleep (REM sleep). Research indicates its significance in shaping a child's memory and brain development, also serving as the stage for dreaming. In newborns, around half of their sleep time is spent in active sleep, whereas adults spend approximately 25% of it in this stage. During REM sleep, a child may exhibit active movements, facial expressions like smiles or frowns, and eye movements under half-open eyelids, giving the impression of potential awakening. Additionally, occasional arm and leg movements might occur.

Drowsiness
In this state, the baby exists in a transitional phase between sleep and wakefulness. It's advisable not to attempt to pick him up or engage him in conversation during this time.

Waking up calmly

The baby appears calm and attentive to his surroundings, with minimal movement. However, he is capable of responding with smiles or facial expressions.

Waking up energetically

The baby is active and appears to be unsettled. He moves his arms and legs, displaying signs as if preparing to cry or yell.

Waking up upset

The baby is upset and cries loudly, and despite your best efforts, you cannot calm him down. This stage may occur in the first weeks after birth but soon passes at the beginning of the third month. Once you have identified the stages of your baby's sleep, you can assist him in organizing his sleep pattern.

Encouraging your baby to form good sleep habits

- Establish a regular routine before sleep, such as bathing and feeding the baby until full, placing him in his crib while playing with him for a short time, and dimming the room. Consistency in this routine will signal the baby that it's time to sleep.
- Introduce a daily routine for the baby, but remain flexible to accommodate your baby's needs and circumstances.
- Gradually encourage your baby to fall asleep on his own without assistance.

- Ensure that the baby's bed is suitable and warm but not excessively so, and avoid using pillows or a soft mattress.
- Prepare everything needed for the night beforehand to avoid disturbing the baby by leaving the room to fetch items.
- Wake the baby for feeding if he has been asleep for an extended period, prioritizing nutrition over prolonged sleep.
- When the baby wakes up crying at night, soothe him without immediately picking him up to avoid reinforcing crying to get attention.
- Avoid smoking near the baby, as exposure to cigarette smoke increases the risk of sudden infant death syndrome (SIDS).
- Encourage naps in the same place where the baby sleeps at night to associate sleep with a particular location.
- Allow the baby a few minutes to settle himself if he cries after waking up, gradually increasing the time before attending to him to encourage self-soothing and independent sleep.

Is it possible to train my baby to differentiate between night and day?

Establishing different habits for day and night can help your baby differentiate between the two. During the day, engage in activities like rocking, playing, singing, and creating a lively atmosphere to stimulate and entertain your baby. However, maintain a quiet environment with dim lights and minimal interaction at night to promote a calm atmosphere conducive to sleep. This distinction will help your baby learn to recognize and adjust to the rhythms of day and night over time.

Dealing with sleep disturbances in babies

Sleep disturbances are common in a baby's early days, but if they persist over a prolonged period, it's essential to investigate several factors:

Temperature in the bedroom

Check the bedroom temperature to ensure it's comfortable, avoiding extremes of warmth or cold. Also, inspect the baby's clothing, as it might contribute to their discomfort if it's too hot.

Is the baby afraid of the dark?

Some children feel uneasy sleeping in complete darkness and may not feel safe. Therefore, having a dim light in the bedroom is beneficial to provide a sense of security for the baby.

Some babies are bothered by excessive light in the bedroom, especially sunlight in the morning.

If sunlight streaming into the room wakes your baby in the morning, consider placing a heavy curtain over the window to block out the light and allow your baby to sleep without disruption.

Noise near the baby

Identifying which sounds bother your baby is essential, as sensitivity to noise differs among infants.

Some may be disturbed by noises like fridges, washing machines, or dripping taps, while others may be bothered by sounds such as doors opening and closing, doorbells, televisions, or children yelling in the house.

Diaper

Ensure the baby's diaper is not wet; if it is, promptly change it.

Check if the baby's clothes are comfortable or not

Loose clothes and socks are more comfortable for the baby and can contribute to peaceful sleep.

Ensure that the baby's crying is not due to hunger

Babies have small stomachs that cannot sustain them for extended periods, so they may wake up when they are hungry.

Messaging your baby

Massage can be incredibly beneficial for babies, as it helps them relax and feel content. Most babies enjoy a massage, especially when accompanied by playful interactions and joking.

Note:

It's common for infants to wake up crying even when none of the usual reasons are present, so there's usually no need to worry about it.

How to deal with early waking

1. Install thick curtains in the baby's room to block daylight.
2. Allow some time before attending to him when he wakes up.
3. To reset his biological clock, keep him awake for an hour before bedtime.

If these methods don't work, you may need to adjust your baby's sleep schedule, as many infants can't sleep until late morning. Adapt to his sleep pattern until he's six months old, as his sleep pattern will likely change by then.

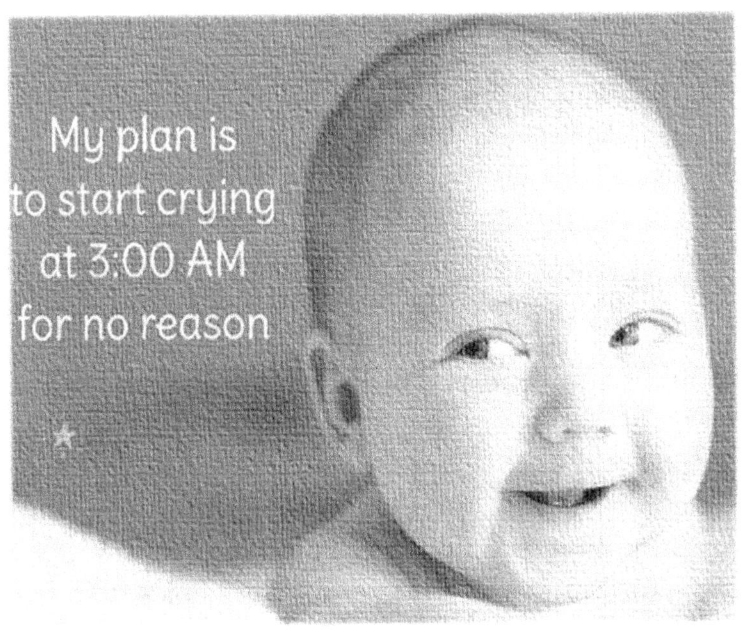

Child development from birth to 3 months

Physical development

Monitoring your baby's development, including his growth, weight, and length/height, is crucial. Keep track of these parameters in his medical records so the doctor can assess his development against average norms. While there's no universal growth pattern for all babies, most fall within certain average ranges, though each baby has a unique rate and pattern of growth.

Rate of weight gain

During the first month of life, infants typically gain between four to seven ounces per week. Subsequently, they usually gain one to two monthly pounds for the following five months. Healthy babies tend to gain around one pound per month from six months to a year. On average, babies gain between seven to 12 pounds (three to five kilograms) from birth to six months; from six months to their first year, they typically gain five to seven pounds (two to three kilograms). The mean growth rate for babies from one year to two years is also around five to seven pounds.

Growth in length/height

From birth to six months, infants typically grow approximately an inch or 2.5 centimeters each month. Afterward, their growth rate slows slightly to around 0.5 inches or a centimeter per month up to their first year of life. On average, babies grow between six to seven inches (15 to 18 cm) in height during the first six months. The normal growth rate is three to four inches (eight to ten cm) from six months to a year. Babies typically grow four to five inches between one year and two years of age (10 to 13 cm).

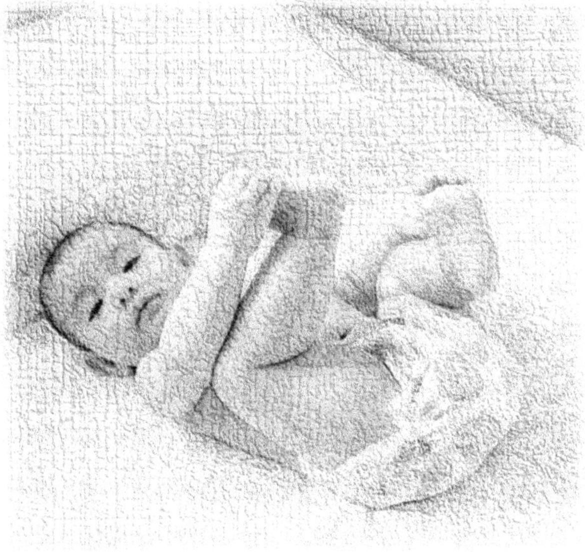

The pattern of developmental milestones
Growth charts for girls

Female Length/height

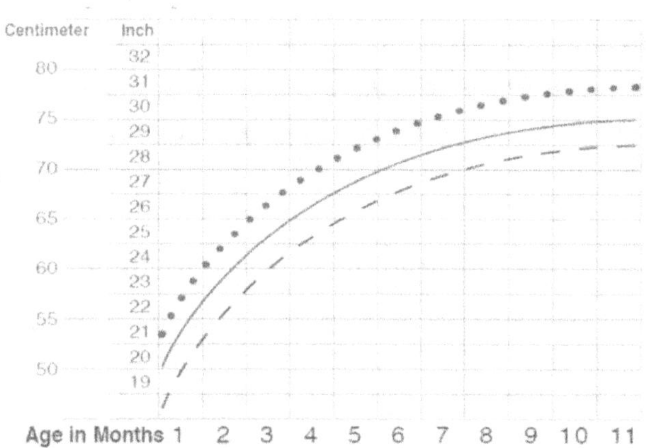

Female Weight

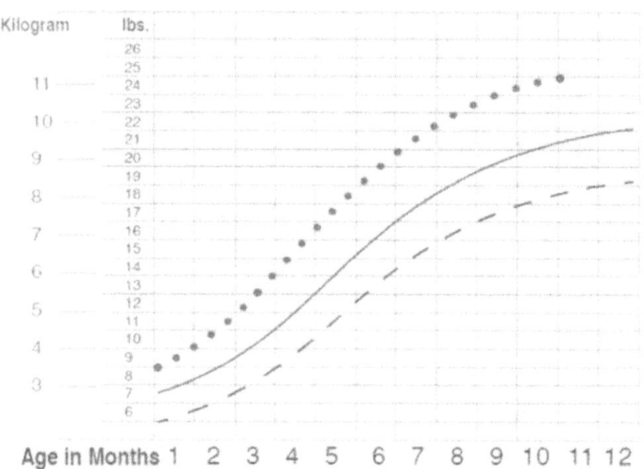

Growth charts for boys

Male Length/height

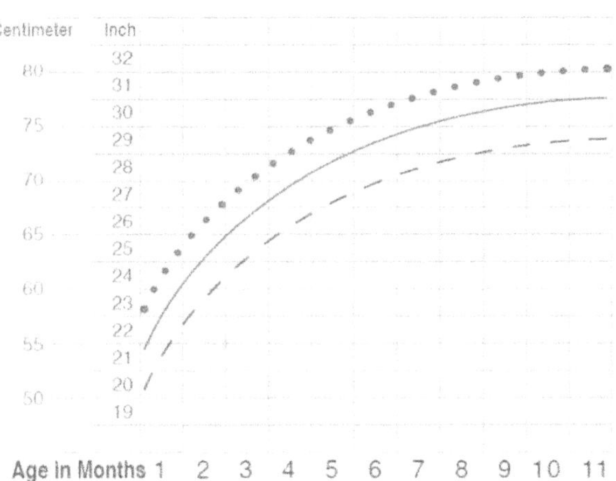

Male Weight

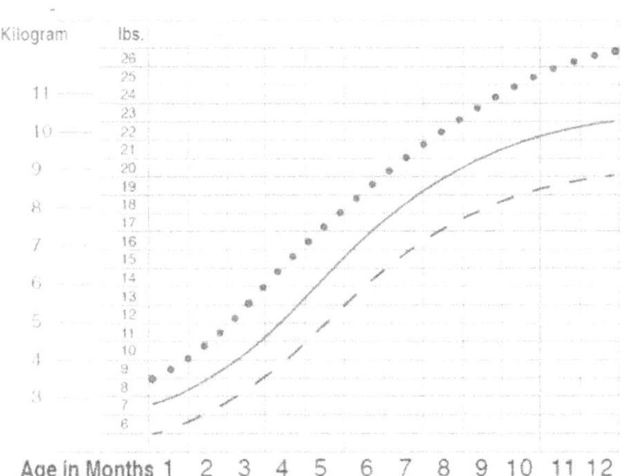

During this month, the baby experiences various physical developments related to the growth of both large and small muscles. Large muscles encompass the torso, neck, legs, and arms, while small muscles involve the hands, feet, and fingers. Hand-eye coordination also improves as a result of the growth of small muscles.

Physical development
The newborn infant lacks control over his movements, which are mainly spontaneous or reflexive. Examples include involuntary smiles, arm movements, and cessation of crying when touched or held by his mother or upon hearing her voice.

- His head may flop backward when attempting to sit him up or dress him.
- When placed on his back, he often assumes a fetal position, drawing his legs toward his tummy and clenching his fists, possibly crying if his legs are stretched out.
- His fists are typically closed or slightly open, and while he may grasp something placed in his hand, he often drops it quickly.
- From birth, the baby starts to explore his limbs, gradually becoming aware of his body parts, beginning with his hands and feet.
- He can track moving objects with his eyes and fixate on them. This ability has been present since birth

for short periods, and now, he can engage in eye-to-eye interaction by focusing on faces and following their movements.

Linguistic development

During the first month, newborns do not make significant linguistic advances. While they may produce random sounds, these noises lack meaning or intentional communication.

Social-emotional development

At this stage, the baby's interaction with those around him is involuntary. He may stop crying when picked up or hearing his mother's voice. Additionally, around one month old, the baby may start making sounds such as gurgling, cooing like a pigeon, or even shouting or mumbling to express his feelings. Responding to him in kind and engaging in face-to-face communication is important.

The second month

Physical development

- The baby opens his eyes more frequently than in the first month, where he spends most of his time with his eyes closed. This may allow you to discern the color of his eyes for the first time.
- The baby shows improved head control, holding his head at the same level as his body when carried.

- When pulled into a sitting position, the baby's head tends to fall backward less than before.
- Movements of the arms and legs remain largely involuntary.
- The baby can now grasp objects longer, although he may still drop them after a minute or two.
- At this stage, your baby's movements become more coordinated, with his previously stiff arm and leg movements becoming softer and more fluid.

Social-emotional development

- The baby begins to interact with the person who talks to him through looking and eye movements as if he is discovering the people around him. His gaze may remain fixed when he hears the voice of someone he loves.
- A warm relationship is formed between the baby and his mother as the infant gazes at his mother.
- During this month, you may enjoy seeing your baby's first intentional smile when you play with him, and he will realize that. This smile is not random or coincidental like in the first month, and it brings great joy to the mother and father. The baby's first smile makes the parents' hearts leap with happiness after many sleepless nights of caring for him without much response.

Linguistic development

Your baby may make some random sounds.

Third month

Physical development
- There is improved coordination between the arms and legs.
- The baby can wave his arms and kick his legs and is physically stronger because the joints of his hips and knees are now more flexible.
- He can put his hands together and spread his fingers but uses his fist to hit dangling things such as suspended toys.
- You will notice that your baby starts to grasp small soft toys, and he may try to bring them to his mouth, but he quickly drops them.
- The movements of his body have changed from involuntary to voluntary movements.
- He turns his head more strongly than in the previous two months.
- He moves his arms and legs on one side with coordination and control.
- He can sit with support.
- Most of the time, his hands stay unclenched.
- He can hold a rattle if his mother puts it in his hand.
- He wants to grab everything he sees.

Social-emotional development ("Hello, I'm here!")

- This month, the baby begins to want to stay with others, and he cries if you leave him on his own, but he calms down and smiles if you pick him up and play with him.
- His sleeping pattern has become smoother and more regular, and now you can get your share of sleep at night.

Linguistic development

The baby produces spontaneous noises that he finds pleasing, such as "gha-gha-gha" and "ah-ah-ah," he shows contentment when you communicate with him using his own vocalizations.

Baby from 4 to 6 months

Feeding your baby
Introducing solid food
Is my baby prepared for solid food?
Your baby is prepared for solid food when:

- He can support his head upright, which is crucial for spoon-feeding.
- His saliva facilitates swallowing solid food.

- With assistance, he can sit up properly. He initially needed support but is progressing to independent sitting in a high chair.
- He can chew food, indicated by the ability to chew and swallow, often accompanied by the appearance of one or two teeth by six months.
- He exhibits increased hunger cues, like waking up at night for additional feeds or seeking more milk.
- His tongue reflex diminishes, typically observed after starting solid food when initially attempting to push food out of the mouth, a normal early response.
- He attains an appropriate weight, with most babies ready for semi-solid food when reaching double their birth weight, often by six months.
- He displays curiosity in your food, showing interest by observing and engaging with it, sometimes attempting to move it from the plate to his mouth.

A few words of advice

1. Avoid introducing solid food too early, as breast milk suffices before four months. The digestive system isn't fully developed, hindering food absorption.
2. don't delay if you sense readiness, as postponing solid food can deprive the baby of essential nutrients like iron and vitamins B and D.
3. Start with tiny portions and introduce solid food gradually to your baby's diet.

4. Respect your baby's food preferences; don't compel him to eat specific foods. If he rejects a food initially, offer alternatives. Reintroduce refused foods later; tastes may change over time.

5. opt for feeding times when your baby is hungry and in a positive mood to ensure better acceptance of solid food.

When should I start to add some solid food along with breast milk?

The World Health Organization suggests introducing complementary foods alongside breast milk between four and six months of age. However, the precise timing can vary and should be determined by a pediatrician, considering the baby's growth rate. If growth is slow, it's advisable to introduce complementary foods earlier, possibly around four months. Conversely, waiting until around five months may be recommended if growth is normal.

Introducing solid food

To start introducing solid foods to your baby, it's recommended to begin with grains like rice, corn, and wheat. Rice is often preferred initially because it's unlikely to cause allergies and can be easily mashed into a purée. Corn can be introduced next after cooking and mashing it. However, wheat should be delayed until around the beginning of the sixth month due to its gluten content, which may trigger allergies in some children.

When offering rice to your baby for the first time, use a small amount on a plastic spoon to avoid discomfort. Initially, your baby may spit out the rice, but with encouragement, they'll gradually accept and enjoy the new food. Adding some breast milk to the rice can help ease the transition.

Avoid adding cow's milk to the rice at this stage as it contains high levels of protein, sodium, potassium, and fats, which can strain the baby's kidneys and digestive system.

It's advisable to offer each new type of food for five or six days before introducing another, allowing the baby to adjust and identifying any potential allergies or sensitivities. Food allergy symptoms may include rash, nausea, stomach pain, diarrhea, itchy skin, shortness of breath, chest pain, swelling of the airways, or anaphylaxis. Stop giving the food and consult your doctor for guidance if you notice any adverse reactions.

A few words of advice

Avoid adding sugar, honey, salt, or spices to the grains, as they can harm your baby at this stage. Gradually increase the amount of food you give your baby until they consume about 2-3 spoons of grains daily. Don't force your baby to eat any food they don't want; you can try again later.

Remember, breast milk remains your baby's primary source of nutrition at this stage. Solid food complements breast milk and should not replace it.

When giving your baby solid food, pay attention to the following:

1. Offer only one type of food in the first five days to ensure your baby isn't allergic and accepts the food.
2. Start with small amounts and gradually increase.
3. Use fresh foods and avoid canned or prepared foods.
4. Ensure your baby is hungry to prevent pushing food out of their mouth.
5. Introduce new foods every few days.
6. Mash or purée foods; avoid foods with texture until later.
7. Offer food on a spoon that allows your baby to take it easily.
8. Dispose of foods in the fridge after one day or longer.
9. Use a small plastic spoon to avoid harming your baby's teeth.
10. Offer familiar foods if your baby is in a bad mood; they may refuse new foods.
11. Prefer natural sugars found in fruits, dates, and raisins over artificial sugars.

12. Wash hands thoroughly and clean utensils and bowls to prevent contamination.
13. Encourage your baby while eating by smiling and playing with them.

Foods that must be avoided during this period

1. Avoid foods with high levels of protein, such as cow's milk. While cow's milk contains some vitamins and minerals like vitamins C and E and iron, it also contains high levels of protein and saturated fats. These substances can be harmful at this stage, as excessive protein intake can lead to antigen-antibody reactions.

What is an antigen-antibody reaction?

The infant's intestines are more sensitive and porous, making it easier for proteins to leak into the bloodstream and interact with the immune system like germs. This can trigger an immune response similar to the body's reaction to pathogens, known as an antigen-antibody reaction.

2. Therefore, it's important to avoid foods containing proteins that may cause allergic reactions, such as legumes (including beans, lentils, and peanuts) and tree nuts, during this period. Additionally, it's essential to keep these foods away from the baby to prevent choking hazards if they are accidentally ingested.

3. Fried or fatty foods
4. Citrus fruits
5. Eggs and their derivatives
6. Onions and garlic
7. Salt, sugar, honey and all kinds of spices

Does solid food change the baby's stools?

When you introduce solid food to your baby, you may notice changes in the color and smell of their stools, which is a natural occurrence. However, if the stool has become excessively solid and is causing discomfort to your child, it's advisable to consult your doctor. In such cases, consider changing the type of food you are giving your baby and incorporating fruits and vegetables into their diet. Additionally, offering the baby some liquids like sips of cooled boiled water or diluted, unsweetened fruit juice can be beneficial.

How can I give my baby more kinds of solid food?

You should introduce new foods gradually, one at a time. Giving your baby some time to adjust to each new taste and texture is essential. This cautious approach allows you to monitor for any potential allergies, such as diarrhea, stomach aches, or skin rashes, that may occur due to introducing a particular food.

Try incorporating a new kind of food every few days, starting with easy fruits and vegetables for infants to digest. For example, you can offer boiled apple and mashed banana, carrots and plums, or sweet potato and white carrot in smooth mixtures by adding boiled and cooled water, breast milk, or artificial milk. You can also try baby rice, wheat, oats, or powdered grains.

It's best to avoid cucumbers, onions, cabbage, broccoli, cauliflower, and similar foods until your baby is one year old, as they can be difficult to digest. Additionally, spinach and beetroot should be avoided because they contain high concentrations of nitrates, which the baby's digestive system may not be able to process effectively before six months.

If your child shows a negative reaction to certain foods, you can try reintroducing them a few days later in the hope that they will accept them.

Feeding your baby in the fifth and six months

At this stage, you can introduce some fruits to your baby's diet, such as pears, apples, bananas, oranges (if they are not acidic), and plums. You can also incorporate other foods like onions and potatoes. Ensure that the food is boiled well and then mashed or puréed. Avoid giving your baby any food that is not puréed. Opt for ripe fruits, which are easier to digest and can be fully puréed.

Offer new foods in small amounts initially to check for any allergies or potential regurgitation. Gradually increase the amount of the new food once you're confident there are no adverse reactions.

You can give your baby diluted fruit juice, such as banana, apple, or peach juice, as long as you dilute it with boiled water first to make it safer for the baby's stomach. Initially, offer the water from a spoon, and later, allow the baby to drink from a cup if they can.

Avoid mixing two kinds of food until you have tried each individually and ensured no allergy. Continue breastfeeding at this stage, as the baby still requires it.

If your baby refuses to let you put the spoon in their mouth, try dipping your finger in the food and then letting them suck it. However, if your baby refuses the spoon, it may be because they do not like that particular food, so try offering them another kind of food instead.

Feeding your baby in the sixth month

- Offer fruit juice, like apple juice, preferably in a cup. If the baby refuses to take the juice from the cup, you can try offering it with a spoon instead.
- Avoid adding salt, sugar, or honey to the baby's food at this stage.
- Begin with a teaspoon of puréed vegetables and gradually increase the amount.
- Avoid mixing two types of vegetables until the baby has tried each one individually.
- Continue breastfeeding, as it remains important for your baby's nutrition and development.

Physical development

- When placed on his tummy, he can lift his head and chest using his forearms to support his body weight.
- He can roll over.
- With assistance, he can sit upright, holding his head steady for a few minutes.
- He shows interest in playing by pulling on his clothes.
- Although he may not be able to pick it up if dropped, he enjoys playing with his rattle for extended periods.
- While lying on his back, he attempts to touch his toes with his hands.
- He picks up objects and puts them in his mouth, showing improved agility and the ability to grasp things firmly.

Social-emotional development

- The baby exhibits hearty laughter during playtime and shows attraction toward colors and movement. He might even smile at his reflection in the mirror. His response to those around him varies based on his comfort level with each individual.
- The baby initiates solo play, engaging with his hands and feet for brief periods, indicating the onset of self-entertainment.

Linguistic development

- Studies indicate that by the fourth month, the baby comprehends the fundamental sounds of his native language. Between the fifth and sixth months, he produces sounds like "mama" and "dada," although he doesn't associate them with specific parents yet.
- He demonstrates the ability to mimic others. When presented with a simple two-letter word like "ma," he attempts to replicate it.
- The baby continues to vocalize sounds he enjoys, such as "wah wah wah," expressing happiness when you echo his sounds.
- Your presence, voice, and facial expressions elicit responses from the baby, often manifesting as kicking legs and waving arms.
- The baby starts to reveal his comfort level with people around him, requiring adequate time to acclimate to unfamiliar faces. He may desire to engage with others, particularly older children who exude energy and enthusiasm when held in your arms.

Five months old

Physical development

- You'll observe your baby becoming capable of grasping the bottle with both hands independently.

- During tummy time, he can significantly lift his head and chest off the ground.
- His hand-eye coordination progresses, allowing him to grasp and hold onto objects and toys.
- He adeptly holds objects between his fingers and explores them by turning them over, often dropping them.
- Your baby demonstrates the capacity to identify small items and moving objects. He begins recognizing objects by glimpsing parts of them, marking the start of games like peek-a-boo that you'll enjoy with him in the upcoming months.

Social-emotional development

- The baby displays hearty laughter and is drawn to colors and movement. He may attempt to mimic the facial expressions of those around him, mirroring laughter and frowns. Additionally, he's starting to exhibit curiosity, exploring his surroundings happily when encountering toys and his bottle.
- Your baby is forming a strong bond with you, evident by his gestures of raising his arms when he wants to be picked up, crying when you leave the room, and even initiating hugs and kisses. Moreover, he's beginning to develop a sense of humor, chuckling at your amusing antics and attempting to elicit laughter from you in return.

Linguistic development

- The baby is experimenting with new sounds, alternating between them, and attempting to mimic sounds he hears.
- He demonstrates awareness of sound direction, turning towards new sounds as they occur. Producing noises with items like a keychain can effectively capture his attention.
- When you speak, the baby observes your mouth movements and endeavors to replicate different sounds, including consonants like "m" and "b."
- At five months old, the baby can recognize his name, which is evident when he responds by turning towards you whenever you call or mention him in conversation.

Six months old

Physical development

- Your baby adeptly grasps small toys with one hand, utilizing all fingers together, and may transfer the toy from one hand to the other. He demonstrates this by holding one block, shifting attention to another, and dropping the first block to pick up a different one.
- He exhibits mobility in all directions, whether lying on his tummy or back.

- With some assistance, he can sit upright and maintain balance.
- He is capable of sitting in a walker.
- When attempting to stand, he doesn't bend his knees.
- He can independently hold his bottle.

Social-emotional development

- By this age, the baby distinguishes familiar faces from strangers and may not readily smile at those he doesn't recognize; he might even cry if approached by them. He strongly attaches to his mother, becoming upset and crying when left alone by her. Additionally, he is capable of hearty laughter and may display preferences for specific toys over others.

Linguistic development

- The baby begins to mimic short words or syllables he has invented and may start picking up other words. He shows attentiveness when his name is mentioned. Additionally, he demonstrates clear abilities to imitate sounds and produces various murmurs and vocalizations.

Nutrition in the seventh and eighth months

- By the seventh month, your baby's jaw movement improves as teeth emerge, indicating readiness for more solid foods like meat, egg yolks, and legumes.
- When introducing meat, ensure it's lean, thoroughly cooked, and finely pureed without added spices or salt. Start with a teaspoon and gradually increase to 2-3 spoonful's daily.
- For legumes, soak them overnight, boil thoroughly, skin them, and then puree.
- Offer only egg yolks, avoiding egg whites.
- Continue breastfeeding alongside introducing solid foods.

Examples of best foods in the seventh and eighth months

Start by offering one food at a time and wait about four days before introducing another to ensure no allergic reactions or sensitivities. Once you've identified safe foods for your baby, you can combine them to create more varied meals.

Cereals

Rice, oatmeal, and barley are commonly among the first solid foods introduced to babies. You can either purchase commercially produced mixes and add previously boiled water following the packaging instructions or make your own by grinding ¼ cup of the grain (avoid "instant" or "quick-cook" oats) in a food processor and then simmering it with a cup of water for about 10 minutes while whisking constantly.

Vegetables

Green beans, carrots, peas, squash, and yams/sweet potatoes are all nutritious options for your baby. Cook or steam the vegetables until tender, then puree them to a smooth consistency before feeding them to your baby.

Fruits

For bananas, mangoes, and avocados, no cooking is required. Simply peel, remove the seed or stone, cut into pieces, and mash or puree them. Papaya may need steaming to break down sugars and fibers, making it easier to digest. Apples, pears, and other similar fruits should be cooked. Peel, remove the core or seeds, cut into pieces, then cook until soft, and mash or puree. Peaches, nectarines, plums, pears, and apricots can be baked, mashed, or pureed after the skins and pits/seeds are removed.

Prunes should be soaked in warm water or steamed until plump and soft, then pureed in a food processor. Be sure to add plenty of water as they become gluey and pasty. Some fruits like melons (8 months) and strawberries (1 year) should be introduced later. Meats and eggs should also be delayed.

If unsure about introducing a certain food, consult a doctor, pediatrician, public health nurse, or reliable print or online resource for advice.

How can I assist my baby to sleep peacefully and comfortably?

Creating a bedtime routine can help your baby sleep well and minimize unnecessary wake-ups. Here are some essential steps:

1. A warm bath can be enjoyable for your baby and help keep them clean.
2. Engage in gentle play with your baby before bedtime to help them relax and feel happy.
3. Ask yourself some questions to address any potential issues that could be affecting your baby's sleep:
   - Is my baby hungry? Consider feeding them if hunger might be a reason for waking up.
   - Is my baby uncomfortable due to a wet diaper or any other discomfort?
   - Is there anything in the environment bothering my baby, such as loud noises or bright lights?
   - Is my baby in a light sleep stage or actively awake?

Addressing these concerns can help create a conducive environment for your baby to sleep deeply through the night.

CRYING

Once your baby reaches six months of age, you'll notice a decrease in crying episodes, and you'll become adept at soothing them due to your growing familiarity with their cues. However, it's important to understand that crying remains a natural part of their communication. Here are several reasons why your baby may continue to cry:

1. **Teething discomfort:** The discomfort associated with teething, as new teeth emerge, can lead to crying.
2. **Introduction of Solid Foods:** Initially, your baby may be unsettled by the introduction of solid foods as they adjust to new tastes and textures. Over time, they will likely grow to enjoy these foods more.
3. **Expression of Needs:** Crying may serve as a way for your baby to communicate desires, such as seeking attention or expressing feelings like loneliness.
4. **Seeking attention:** Your baby may cry to indicate a desire for more attention, especially if they feel their caregiver's focus has shifted away.
5. **Boredom:** Crying may occur when your baby feels bored or lacks stimulation due to distractions from household tasks. Providing age-appropriate toys can help keep them engaged.
6. **Exploration and Safety:** As your baby becomes more mobile around their first year, they may cry

due to minor accidents or bumps while exploring their surroundings. Ensuring a safe environment is essential to prevent injuries.

Understanding these factors can help you respond to your baby's needs effectively and provide them with comfort and reassurance during moments of distress.

General changes at this stage (7-12 months)

Teething

Many mothers mistakenly believe that their baby's teeth begin to appear after birth, but tooth development starts as early as the fifth month of gestation. These first teeth, known as milk teeth, emerge around the sixth month of the baby's life and continue to do so until they are around two and a half years old.

Milk teeth consist of four front teeth, four molars, and two canines in each jaw. Dental care for the baby should commence as early as the fourth month of pregnancy, with the mother's diet playing a crucial role in tooth formation.

Typically, teeth emerge first in the lower jaw before appearing in the upper jaw, although the order may vary from one child to another. If a baby's teeth do not appear by the end of their first year, it is advisable to seek guidance from a healthcare professional.

Common signs of teething

1. The gums become inflamed and swollen.
2. Excessive drooling and flushed cheeks are common.
3. A mild cough may be present.
4. The baby seeks to alleviate discomfort by biting on objects.
5. Initial tooth eruption may cause discomfort and increased drooling.
6. Irritability and changes in temperament can occur.
7. The baby may chew on solid items and suck on fingers for relief.

Some mothers believe teething is linked to symptoms like diarrhea, fever, and chest infections. However, there's no direct correlation between these symptoms and teething. Mothers must consult a doctor if their baby experiences such symptoms, even if they coincide with teething.

Taking care of the baby's teeth during and after the teething stage

Caring for milk teeth is crucial as they are more susceptible to damage than permanent teeth, and neglecting them could impact the subsequent teeth. To ensure proper care:

- Provide the baby with foods rich in nutrients essential for proper tooth development, such as calcium and vitamin D.
- Continue breastfeeding, as the mother's milk is rich in calcium, vital for building the child's teeth.
- Clean the baby's teeth with a soft brush, using gentle up-and-down motions, ensuring not to injure the gums.

Do pacifiers and teething rings help with teething?

Many mothers consider pacifiers and finger-sucking beneficial during teething, but in reality, pacifiers can do more harm than good due to various reasons:

- Pacifiers can adversely affect the baby's jaw and milk teeth.
- They are prone to contamination, introducing germs into the baby's mouth, potentially leading to diseases.
- Children using pacifiers are more susceptible to crooked teeth and bite problems.

Finger Sucking

Finger-sucking is a common habit in children, often starting soon after birth and lasting until they are weaned and sometimes even continuing after weaning. This behavior may stem from anxiety or a longing for the mother's breast after weaning. It's a natural part of childhood, as infants rely on sucking for comfort from the earliest stages of life. In such cases, it's advisable for mothers not to scold the child for this habit, as it could exacerbate feelings of anxiety.

Instead, continuing breastfeeding for up to two years, if possible, can help reduce the need for finger-sucking. If the habit persists, it typically fades away once the child is fully weaned.

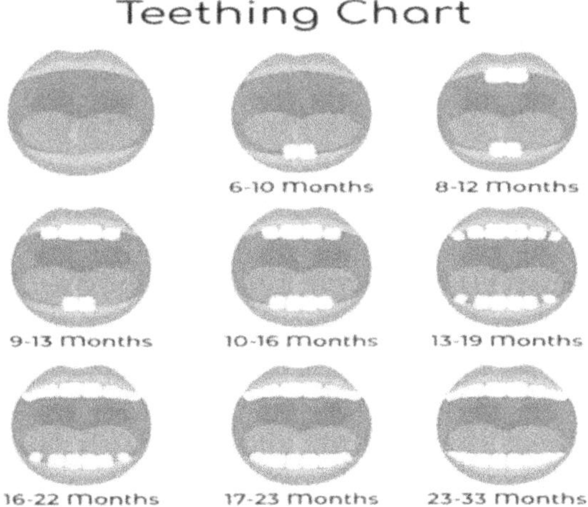

Reducing the pain of teething
If your baby is experiencing discomfort due to teething, it's important to offer comfort and alleviate their pain using one of the following methods:

- Gently massage the gum with your finger.
- Apply sugar-free teething gel to the affected area to ease the pain as the tooth emerges.

- Give your baby plenty of cold drinks to help numb the area.
- Offer a rubber teething ring for them to chew on; refrigerating it beforehand can enhance its soothing effect.
- Consider using teething remedies like chamomile drops.
- If a rash develops under the baby's chin due to drooling, apply Vaseline to soothe the affected area.

When will my baby start remembering things?

Memory is the mental faculty through which individuals can recall past or present images, sounds, and events. It serves as a connection between the past and the present, with children beginning to develop this ability at an early age. By the second month, infants exhibit signs of remembering people and simple actions, although their memory capacity is limited during this stage.

Recognition memory, which involves the child's ability to identify familiar people and objects, becomes more pronounced as the child grows.

Newborns can recognize their mother's voice shortly after birth, having become accustomed to hearing it in the womb, and breastfeeding babies can identify their mother's smell within a week. Over time, infants start to recognize familiar faces, such as their parents.

Retrieval and recall abilities emerge between six months and one year, allowing the child to remember specific experiences. As their memory strengthens, children become more adept at recalling information that interests them or occurs frequently in their environment. They may remember the location of their toys or imitate actions observed in the past week, signaling their understanding of routine activities like meals or bedtime.

As children grow older, their memory capacity expands, enabling them to store various images. Studies have shown that four-year-old children can recall images presented briefly, demonstrating an average accuracy rate of 80%. However, long-term memory and memory of specific events typically develop between fourteen and eighteen months of age.

Research on children aged five to six has revealed their ability to remember words, movements, images, and meanings. They exhibit better recall for clear words and phrases than ambiguous ones and recognize missing elements in pictures. These findings illustrate the progression of memory capabilities and cognitive development as children age.

The seventh month

Physical development

- The baby demonstrates vigorous limb movements, kicking and pushing objects with his feet and mastering the skill of rolling over from his stomach onto his back and vice versa.
- He attempts to pull himself into a standing position but has not yet achieved it.

- He can grasp onto objects with both hands for an extended period.
- He shows increased joy during playtime and can manage multiple toys simultaneously.
- He can lift his upper body and even begin crawling backward.
- When placed in a sitting position, he displays steady head control.

Social-emotional development

- The baby shows distress when strangers try to pick him up; he can now distinguish his mother, father, and other family members. He enjoys toys that produce gentle sounds.

Linguistic development

- The baby listens attentively to the speech of those around him and may start producing unique sounds consisting of three syllables, like "da-da-da" or "ba-ba-ba."

The eight-month

Physical development

- Toddlers can sit up unassisted at this stage.
- Infants of this age can crawl.
- children can roll onto their backs when placed on their stomachs.

- Your baby might be capable of standing up, relying on furniture for support.
- Assistance may be needed for the baby to sit down from standing.
- Your baby will demonstrate the ability to pick up small objects.
- The baby can move their knees and wave their arms while standing.

Linguistic development

- The baby can recognize specific sounds, like a cat's "meow" or a train's "choo-choo."
- He begins comprehending the meanings of "no" and "yes."
- When his name is called, he turns around; if your child doesn't respond to sounds or his name, consult a doctor.

Social-emotional development

- The baby enjoys being the center of attention within the family.
- He becomes anxious when surrounded by strangers, particularly when tired, upset, or his mother is not nearby, showing signs of worry. Although it's tough to see your child upset, allowing him to experience this briefly and returning reassures him of your consistent presence, fostering confidence and social skills.

- He prefers being held by his parents when strangers are present.
- His interest lies more in his toys.
- The baby finds joy when you sit with him, draw, and share short stories.
- He attempts to mimic his parents, emphasizing the importance of a positive example.
- At this stage, most children explore objects through shaking, hitting, dropping, and throwing before returning to their tendency to put things in their mouths.
- The child delights in looking at himself in a mirror.

The ninth month

Physical development

- At this stage, the baby attempts to stand without support from furniture. Achieving this milestone brings him great joy.
- The child has developed the ability to transition from standing to sitting.
- With support, he can walk.
- He begins to manipulate toy buttons with his fingers.
- Some children may show signs of being able to feed themselves with a spoon.
- You'll observe his ability to sit, stand, and engage in purposeful seated movements.
- He may attempt to crawl upstairs.

- When someone waves bye-bye to him, he can reciprocate the gesture.

Linguistic development

- You might hear him clearly say "Mama" for the first time.
- The child often repeats various words and sounds, although he doesn't grasp their meanings yet.
- He begins comprehending "no" and may enjoy doing things you've forbidden.

Social-emotional development

- The child can now communicate his needs and desires more effectively. If you try to remove a toy he likes, he may express objection and yell.
- He better understands height and space, possibly showing fear of elevated places.
- The child exhibits increased attachment to his mother. If she leaves him with strangers or steps away, he may become upset, yelling, or crying for an extended period.

The tenth month

Physical development

- He may achieve standing independently at this stage.
- He navigates by holding onto furniture for support.

- He climbs onto chairs and ascends stairs.
- He might develop the ability to drink from a cup.
- He transfers toys between his hands and throws them forcefully.
- At this age, he engages with colored blocks during play.

Linguistic development

- He comprehends more words.
- He may vocalize simple words with meaning, so continue conversing with your child even if it seems trivial at times. It's an excellent method to nurture his language skills. When he vocalizes a string of unintelligible words, respond with, "Really? How nice." You'll notice he smiles and continues talking, and soon, you'll recognize some understandable words or gestures alongside other forms of communication like pointing or babbling.

Social-emotional development

- He comprehends the meaning of play and enjoys engaging with you. A game like "Peek-a-boo" is enjoyable for your child, where you cover your face and ask, "Where am I?" then reveal your face and say, "Here I am!"
- At this stage, your child's social tendencies become evident. He might be affectionate, smiling broadly

at everyone, or he might be more reserved, hiding his face when greeted by strangers.

- He may mimic actions and sounds to attract your attention and wave goodbye as you leave.
- Additionally, the child becomes more capable of expressing emotions such as happiness, joy, sadness, and anxiety.
- He can wave goodbye, clap his hands, and move his body.
- Furthermore, he can respond to some questions posed to him. For example, if asked, "Where is Baba?" he may point to him.

The eleventh month

Physical development

- He can stand independently and bend down while standing.
- He is capable of climbing stairs.
- He can drink from a cup.
- He can squat.
- He crawls energetically forward and may even crawl while carrying a toy.

Linguistic development

- At this stage, your child can say some words or make some sounds, and he may even use some words correctly, but most of his words are still repeated without full understanding.

- He can imitate the pronunciation and tone of some words just as he imitates actions. He can respond to simple requests such as, "Please give me the ball" or "Give me a spoon." Help him learn by giving him simple instructions that are easy to follow.

Social-emotional development

- This month is a period of exploration for your child. He will discover cupboards, drawers, bags, toy boxes, and kitchen tools.
- Your child enjoys looking at books and turning the pages, often having a favorite he returns to frequently.
- He mimics the movements of older children.
- At this age, your child can distinguish between actions that please you and those that upset you, as well as between obedience and disobedience. If he doesn't follow your instructions, it may be deliberate.
- It's a time for setting boundaries. While you shouldn't be harsh, it's important to establish limits. For instance, if he wants a second cupcake, gently refuse. If he pulls the cat's tail, gently correct him, explaining why it's wrong and how to treat the cat gently.
- Understand that what may appear as disobedience is often just natural curiosity and a desire to

explore. It's your role to guide and protect him while he learns about the world.

- Your child may object if anyone takes something from his hand, even if it doesn't belong to him.

The twelfth month

Physical development

- Some children achieve walking milestones at this age.
- At this stage, crawling becomes faster for the child.
- Falling frequently is common when a child is learning to walk.
- Despite being able to walk, the child may still prefer crawling.
- He can search for a lost toy.
- Attempts to remove clothing may occur.
- He engages in play with cans and attempts to open them.
- Climbing on furniture is a new exploration at this age.

Linguistic development

- Now, he can clearly articulate three or four words, such as Baba, Mama, and Dada.
- He comprehends the meaning of simple commands like "Go ahead," "come here," "look," "no," and "go."

- Encourage your child to link objects with their names. The more you do this, the more extensive his vocabulary will become. Engage in conversation with your child, labeling everything; even count the stairs as you climb them. Introduce him to the store's names of fruits, vegetables, and colors. Additionally, read picture books together and encourage him to identify or name familiar objects. Occasionally, offer choices like asking if he prefers the red or blue socks or if he wants to play with the blocks or the rings. Your child might not respond immediately, or he might pleasantly surprise you.

Social-emotional development

- At this stage, your child will assert his position among his siblings and develop greater self-reliance.
- He enjoys tossing objects onto the ground and may swap toys frequently.
- Collecting items in containers and then emptying them out becomes a favorite activity, including pots and pans. He might stack pans or put smaller items inside larger ones to hear the noises they make.
- He shows more interest in playing with peers.
- He becomes attuned to the emotions of others, noticing if his mother is happy or upset.
- The one-year-old is akin to a teenager entering adolescence; he desires independence and freedom of movement.

- Your child starts attempting to fit small objects into corresponding holes and may experiment with inserting items into his nose.

Physical development

- By the thirteenth month, most children can walk without assistance, albeit unsteadily, often relying on furniture for support. What's important is their newfound ability to move independently, no longer requiring constant carrying.
- They may ascend stairs on their hands and knees, exploring their newfound mobility and spatial awareness.
- Climbing into their crib marks another milestone, demonstrating their growing physical capabilities and autonomy.
- Growth rate and food intake tend to slow down at this stage compared to earlier phases. While growth during the first year is rapid, it begins to taper off between the first and second birthdays.
- Children can engage with picture books, turn pages, and show interest in visual stimuli, indicating cognitive development.
- Basic problem-solving skills emerge as they build small towers with blocks.

- Exploring their environment, they may attempt to grasp and turn doorknobs, showing curiosity and a desire for independence.

Linguistic development

- Towards the end of the fifteenth month, the child's vocabulary expands to around 6 words, marking a significant linguistic development.
- They start grasping simple instructions like "Take," "Come," and "Go," demonstrating early language comprehension.
- Recognizing body parts becomes apparent as they learn the names of different body parts, enhancing their cognitive understanding.
- Attempting to mimic the words of others shows their growing language acquisition skills and eagerness to communicate.

Social-emotional development

- With newfound mobility, your child's curiosity leads them wherever their feet take them.
- As their walking skills advance, so does their manual dexterity.
- By thirteen months, most children can pick up blocks and place them in a box; some even start scribbling.
- Your child might be able to hold a spoon, showing progress in self-feeding.

- Playtime involves experimentation, like testing what happens when throwing a cup or dipping fingers in food.
- Developing bladder control emerges, with some children beginning to indicate when to urinate.
- Picture books captivate them, fostering early literacy skills.
- They observe and imitate adult actions.
- Persistently exploring desires, often challenging safety boundaries, requires continuous supervision.
- They're refining spoon skills while exploring textures and consequences of actions.
- Recognizing themselves in the mirror, they start seeing themselves as distinct individuals, even trying to kiss their reflection.
- "No" becomes a frequently used word, asserting independence in decision-making.

sixteen to eighteen months

Physical development

- Enhanced walking skills emerge, with improved balance and stronger trunk muscles allowing for standing, turning, bending, and stopping without toppling.
- Increased agility enables the child to move swiftly, run, and execute two-footed jumps.

- Squatting from a standing position becomes effortless for the child.
- Hand coordination progresses as the child adeptly grasps food items and can choose to hold them or release them.
- Hand preference becomes apparent, potentially revealing the child's dominant hand, often around this age.
- Gesturing while speaking becomes a common communication trait.
- Holding a pen and scribbling signifies fine motor skill development.
- Exploring drawers and engaging with the contents become favorite activities, showcasing the child's growing curiosity and manual dexterity.

Linguistic development

- Vocabulary expands to around 10 words, marking progress in language development.
- Comprehension extends beyond spoken words, with the child understanding more words than he can verbally express.
- Two-word sentences emerge, showcasing the child's ability to combine words to convey simple ideas.
- Introduction of basic spatial concepts through gestures, such as indicating "above" or "below," demonstrates cognitive growth and symbolic understanding.

Social-emotional development

- Tantrums are common as your toddler struggles to manage overwhelming emotions. Be patient and understanding during these episodes.
- Your child begins to categorize and differentiate between toys, understanding similarities and differences.
- Picky eating habits may emerge, with your child showing preferences for certain foods and rejecting others.
- Curiosity blossoms at this stage, with your child eager to explore and learn about the world.
- Scribbling and drawing lines become favorite activities, fostering creativity and fine motor skills.
- Minor behavioral issues like jealousy and stubbornness may arise as your child asserts independence.
- Mood swings and unpredictability are typical as your child navigates complex emotions.
- Fear of strangers diminishes as your child grows more comfortable with unfamiliar faces.
- Affection for toys grows as your child expresses love for their favorite playthings.
- Increased understanding of cause and effect lets your child anticipate outcomes and problem-solve creatively.

- Play with dolls becomes more imaginative, with your child engaging in caregiving behaviors like feeding and grooming.
- Active play, such as running and ball games, brings joy and excitement, especially with interaction from caregivers.

Nineteen to twenty-four months

Physical development

- Your child demonstrates soccer skills by kicking the ball with one foot and chasing after it.
- Engaging in active play, he enjoys running, playing soccer, and seeking hiding spots behind furniture.
- Improved balance, agility, and stair-climbing abilities indicate growing physical coordination.
- Steady height and weight gain reflect healthy growth and development.
- Responding to music, he moves his whole body in rhythm, showing increased musical engagement.
- Enhanced hand and finger coordination and better eye control enable more precise movements.
- He participates in various games that require motor, visual, and mental skills, showcasing his growing abilities in multiple areas.

Linguistic development

- With an expanded vocabulary, the child knows between twenty and fifty words.
- He converses with both parents, forming sentences using his growing vocabulary.
- A common phrase he frequently utters is "What is that?" reflecting his heightened curiosity, which is typical for this developmental stage.
- He can respond to simple questions like "Where is your brother?", "What did you eat?" and "Where is the toy?" indicate his ability to understand and communicate basic information.

Social-emotional development

- At this stage, your toddler becomes more aware of gender differences.
- Your daughter may start imitating women's behavior while your son mimics men's actions. However, it's normal for children to imitate both sexes, so don't be surprised if your son imitates women or your daughter imitates men.
- Your toddler begins to recognize when things don't make sense to adults and may laugh at absurdities, such as calling a giraffe a donkey or mistaking his sister for his brother.
- Toddlers are naturally curious, including about their genitals. Just as they explored their fingers and toes earlier, they may now explore their

genitalia. If your child does this in front of others, calmly explain it's inappropriate.

- The child still craves attention and seeks to be the center of it.
- He may display various feelings and behaviors, including violence, biting, stubbornness, jealousy, anger, and fear of certain things.
- He demonstrates love towards his parents and loved ones, calling them by their names.
- At 21 months, your child may show interest in tidying up, organizing, and helping with household chores. He may also start dressing, washing and drying his hands, and brushing his teeth with minimal assistance.
- Your child begins to assert his independence, taking care of some of his affairs, which indicates his growing sense of security. Respect his preferences and interests, and offer clear guidance on behaviors that are not negotiable for safety reasons.
- You may notice your child showing a preference for one hand over the other, which is typically genetic.
- Transition your child to a big bed before he can climb out of the crib independently. Involve him in the process by letting him choose his bed and sheets. Be patient during the adjustment period, as he may initially struggle with the change.
- Your child starts to empathize with others' emotions. For example, he may feel sad when he

sees another child hurt or disturbed when witnessing parental arguments.

- His memory and ability to form mental images improve, and he may express hostility towards those who frustrate him.

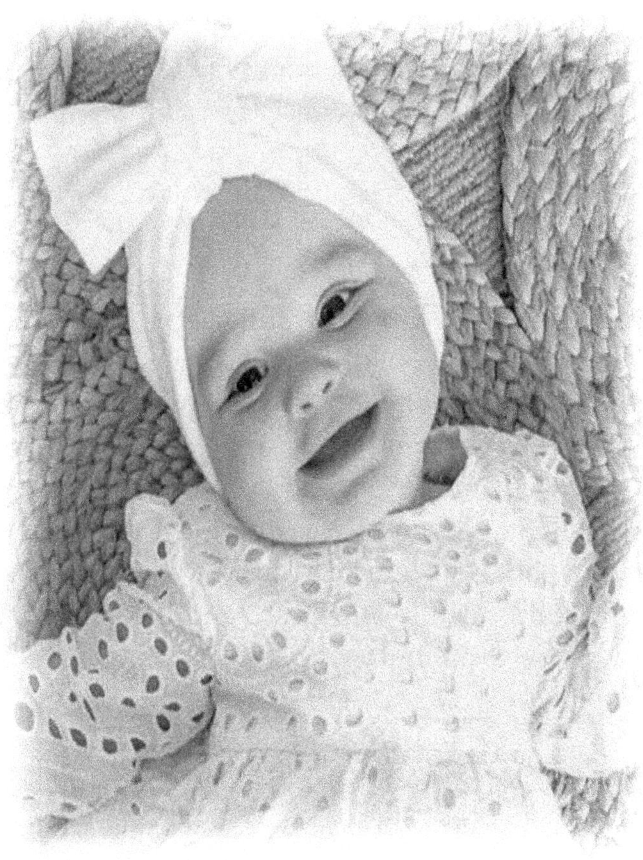

As your child's mobility expands, so does his exposure to potential dangers while exploring various areas of the house, including the kitchen, bedroom, garden, and beyond. Therefore, each time he acquires a new skill, it necessitates implementing additional measures and precautions to ensure his safety.

Necessary measures to keep your child safe

- Carefully look around your home, considering things from your child's perspective. Sit beside your child on the floor to identify potential hazards that may catch his attention or curiosity, and take steps to mitigate any associated risks.
- Reevaluate the layout and organization of items within your home to create a safer environment for your child. Arrange furniture and belongings in a way that minimizes potential dangers and promotes safety.
- Stay vigilant and attentive to your child's growth and development, both physically and mentally. As he reaches new milestones such as crawling, walking, and standing, be aware of the evolving risks he may encounter and adapt your safety measures accordingly.

Safety in the kitchen is paramount, especially with curious little ones around. Here are some precautions to help keep your child safe:

- Store kitchen utensils away from the edge of counters where your child can't reach them.
- Avoid carrying your child while cooking or preparing food.
- Keep sharp objects like knives, forks, and spoons out of your child's reach.
- Store cleaning solutions, soaps, and other liquids in high cabinets.
- Keep plastic bags out of reach to prevent suffocation hazards.
- Remove electrical appliance plugs from sockets to prevent accidents.
- Ensure hot liquids like tea and coffee are kept away from your child.
- Dispose of leftover milk promptly to prevent accidental ingestion.
- Avoid using tablecloths your child could pull, causing items to fall.
- Keep electrical appliances away from water sources and disconnect them when not in use.
- Keep the kitchen floor dry and free of slippery substances.

- Store matches in a secure location inaccessible to your child.
- Place dangerous items like knives in high places or locked cabinets as your child explores drawers.
- Secure appliances like the fridge, washing machine, and dryer to prevent access that could lead to accidents.

Safety measures in the bathroom

Bath time safety is crucial to protect your child from accidents. Here are some important tips:

- Prepare everything you need for the bath to avoid leaving the bathroom while your child is in the tub.
- Never leave your child unattended in the bathtub, even for a moment. Always take them with you if you must leave the bathroom.
- Ensure all vessels and the bathtub are emptied of water immediately after use.
- Be cautious of the toilet, as most drowning incidents occur when a child leans over it and falls in. Keep the toilet lid closed at all times.
- Consider installing a toilet seat lock for added safety.
- Always check the water temperature with a thermometer before bathing your baby. Aim for around 37°C, and add cold water first before adjusting with hot water.

- Keep the bathroom door closed to prevent your child from accessing the bathroom unsupervised and encountering potential hazards.

Keeping your baby safe in the bedroom

Ensuring a safe sleeping environment for your baby is essential. Here are some important guidelines to follow:

- Provide a separate crib for your baby to reduce the risk of accidental suffocation, especially if you tend to sleep deeply.
- Maintain a suitable temperature in the bedroom to keep your baby comfortable.
- Avoid leaving electrical or gas heaters on in the child's room while sleeping.
- Refrain from placing a pillow in your baby's crib. If needed, elevate the mattress instead.
- Do not leave a bottle in your baby's mouth while they sleep to prevent choking hazards.
- Always place your newborn on their back to sleep to reduce the risk of SIDS.
- Keep solid or hard toys away from your child's sleeping area to prevent injuries.
- Regularly monitor your child's growth and development to ensure their safety in the crib.
- Store sharp utensils and dangerous objects in locked drawers to prevent access by curious hands.

- Use stable and sturdy furniture in your child's bedroom to avoid tipping hazards.
- Opt for furniture with rounded edges and corners to minimize the risk of injury from collisions.

Keeping your baby safe in the house:

general tips

Ensuring your baby's safety in various areas of the house and garden is crucial. Here are some additional precautions to take:

In the House:

- Never leave your baby alone in a room with lit fires, stoves, or desk fans.
- Avoid smoking cigarettes in front of your child to prevent exposure to harm and the potential for imitation.
- Secure and lock windows to prevent falls and injuries.
- Remove ropes and strings from blinds and curtains to prevent strangulation hazards.
- Keep tables free of glass and metal objects, and avoid using tablecloths that hang down.
- Avoid leaving small items within reach that could pose a choking hazard.
- Cover electrical outlets with protective covers to prevent the child from inserting objects.

- Install rubber protectors on sharp edges and corners to minimize injuries from collisions.
- Keep chairs or climbable objects away from windows to prevent falls.
- Supervise your baby when using a walker to prevent accidents.
- Install safety gates at the top and bottom of stairs to prevent falls.

In the Garden:

- Avoid letting your child play in areas where insecticides have been used.
- Ensure that outdoor furniture has no sharp edges or corners.
- Supervise interactions with pets, as animals may behave unpredictably.
- Empty paddling pools after use to prevent drowning hazards.
- Store garden tools, insecticides, and harmful plants in a secure area.
- Cover the garden with grass or sand to cushion falls.
- Supervise your child at all times outdoors and teach them not to eat harmful substances like sand and weeds.

Keeping your baby safe in the car

Car safety for children is paramount, and there are specific precautions to follow:

- Use seats appropriate for the child's weight and age, ensuring the seat belt fits comfortably and securely around them. Professional installation is recommended.

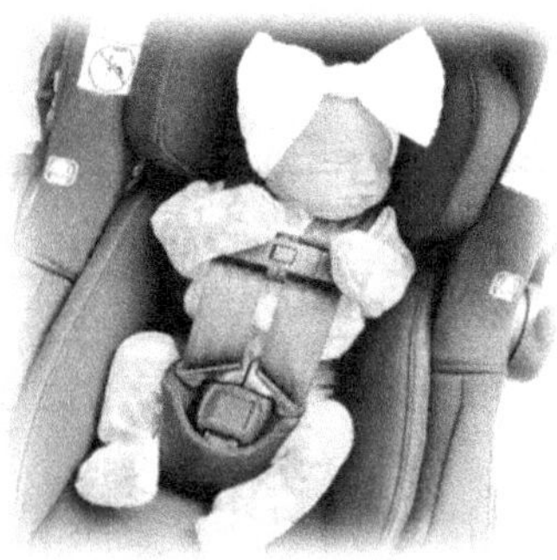

Note: In some regions, there's a misconception that it's safer for a child to sit on a parent's lap in the car. However, this is more dangerous in the event of a crash, as the child is at risk of being crushed between the adult and the dashboard.

- Place newborn car seats on the back seat, facing backward, for added safety.
- Ensure all car doors are properly closed, and consider using central locking if available.
- Never leave newborns unattended in the car.

- When removing the child from the car, do so on the side closest to the sidewalk for added safety.
- Use appropriate shades or coverings to Protect the child from harmful sun rays while in the car.

Important note for fathers and mothers

Before driving the car, always ensure no children are under or near it. Some children, especially those who have recently learned to walk, may gravitate towards sitting under the car or near its tires, posing a serious risk of injury.

Keeping children safe when taking them outside

- Always keep a firm grip on your child's hand whenever you're out. If you can't bring the stroller into a location, either take your child out of the stroller or avoid entering that place altogether.
- If you lose sight of your child outside the house, contact the nearest police station immediately.
- Gradually teach your child, without causing fear, about the importance of not wandering off alone and not going with anyone who tries to persuade them to go somewhere.
- Avoid crossing streets with high-speed traffic while pushing a stroller, as drivers may not notice you have a child with you. go for designated pedestrian crossings whenever possible to ensure safety.

Feeding your child

By the beginning of the ninth month, your child will likely have adapted to most types of food, allowing you to incorporate some of the family's meals into their diet, provided they are free of spices, salt, and sugar.

From the start of the tenth month until around eighteen months old, your child will become more accustomed to eating meals with the family. However, it's important to still serve the child's food separately and ensure it remains free of spices and salt. You can achieve this by setting aside a portion of rice, meat, and vegetables before seasoning with spices or salt for yourself and your partner.

When is the right time to stop breastfeeding?

In many Western nations, mothers typically cease breastfeeding once their child reaches six months of age. It's uncommon to find mothers who breastfeed beyond this timeframe. However, I'm afraid I have to disagree with this trend because I believe that children still benefit from breast milk after the six-month mark. In my view, preparations to discontinue breastfeeding should commence around the beginning of the second half of the child's second year, with breastfeeding coming to a complete halt by the end of that year. By this stage, the child is typically ready to join the family for meals.

But stopping breastfeeding must be done gradually and slowly

Take the   following   steps:

- Discontinue the mid-morning breastfeeding session and offer a cup of water instead.
- Eventually, replace the lunchtime breastfeeding session with solid food.
- After three days, introduce a meal of fresh fruit and water in place of the evening breastfeeding session.
- Following this, occasional breastfeeding sessions may still occur at different times. Gradually reduce these by engaging the child in other activities when they seek to breastfeed. Encourage your partner to spend time with the child outdoors or take them for a walk. Over time, breastfeeding will cease entirely.

Taking care of milk teeth

Causes of cavities in milk teeth

- Excessive intake of processed sugar is the primary cause of cavities in baby teeth.
- Drinking carbonated beverages can contribute to tooth decay.

- Consuming large quantities of cookies, chocolate, and sticky sweets is also a factor.
- Inadequate attention to breastfeeding can affect dental health.
- An imbalanced diet lacking essential nutrients like iron, calcium, and phosphorus may lead to tooth problems.
- Neglecting to properly clean the child's teeth and leaving food particles between them can contribute to cavities.

Protection against cavities in milk teeth

- It's important to shield your child from consuming hidden sugars like sucrose, glucose, lactose, and fructose in various sources.
- Sugar's impact is mitigated when consumed during meals, as fats help protect teeth, and saliva aids in cleaning sugar from tooth surfaces and restoring enamel.
- Encourage your child to choose healthy meals and avoid sticky sweets, dried fruits, and mint-flavored chewing gum, which prolongs sugar exposure due to their viscosity.
- Offering sugar-free gum in moderation can promote saliva production.
- Substitute fizzy drinks containing citric and phosphoric acids with milk or diluted fruit juice.

- Regular dental checkups are crucial to detect and address potential cavities in your child's teeth and to receive guidance on oral care practices.

When should the child move from the crib to a bed?

The appropriate time to transition the child from a crib to a bed is when they can climb out of the crib, posing a risk of falling. Additionally, if the child becomes upset or feels constrained in the crib, signaling a need for more freedom, it's time to consider moving them to a regular bed. This transition typically occurs around the age of two years or older.

Pampering the child

Will pampering my child lead to spoiling him?

Is it harmful to constantly fulfill all of my child's desires?

Will being lenient with my child result in him having a weak personality?

These concerns cross the minds of many mothers.

In reality, the act of spoiling children unfolds in two phases:

Pampering the baby in the first few months of life

During this phase, the mother shouldn't worry about spoiling her child with excessive pampering.
If the baby cries or struggles to sleep, picking him up, walking with him, cuddling him, and providing comfort as needed is important. This could be because the baby is experiencing discomfort, colic, or tension, requiring extra support and care.

By comforting the child, distracting him, and gently massaging his tummy while holding him, it's possible to alleviate some of his discomfort and tension, even if only temporarily. Pampering the baby during this period helps instill confidence and security in his surroundings.

Pampering the baby once he is past the age of 6 to 9 months

At this stage, it's important to recognize the necessity of withholding certain things from the child if it's in their best interest. This shouldn't be seen as cruel but rather as understanding what's best for the child.

For instance, a mother who constantly carries her child may find it challenging to accomplish household tasks when the child becomes accustomed to constant attention and demands it persistently.

Similarly, if a child consistently requests certain foods like candy or chips, granting these requests excessively can lead to spoiled behavior.

Dr. Azeezah al-Sayyid, a professor of psychology, warns against excessive pampering, which can lead to the child developing an unstable character and being unable to cope with pressure or delays in fulfilling desires.

This may result in selfishness, difficulty forming social relationships, and challenges in adhering to rules and regulations in the future.

Inconsistent parenting, alternating between strictness and leniency, can confuse the child. Parents must agree on a unified approach to avoid confusion for the child.

Excessive strictness can breed hostility and hinder successful relationships, as it may cause the child to resent authority. Moreover, parents resorting to anger, hitting, or derogatory language can make the child feel unsafe and insecure.

While adults may justify strictness as an attempt to instill ideal behavior, it often leads to apathy in the child rather than compliance.

Aggression in children – causes and remedy

Aggression is defined as behavior that inflicts harm on others. According to Berkowitz, aggression arises from intense frustration stemming from negative emotions.

The following are characteristics of an aggressive child:

- Difficulty expressing their feelings
- Resistance to criticism
- Tendency towards introversion and frustration
- Emotional immaturity

Imitation of aggressive behavior that he sees
For instance, aggression can stem from interactions with one's father, siblings, or mother. Research indicates that aggressive behavior exhibited by parents significantly influences the emergence of aggression in their children.

Family disputes
Research conducted by Kokus in 1979-1980 revealed a correlation between parental divorce and the onset of aggressive behavior in children. This connection is attributed to the pressure and conflict within the home

environment, which can provoke such negative reactions in children.

Watching violent scenes on television

Alternatively, exposure to computer games centered around themes of combat, violence, and aggression can also contribute to the development of aggressive behavior in children.

Differences in the way children in the same family are treated

Parents sometimes favor a child perceived as good-looking, intelligent, or obedient while treating a less attractive, slower, or more stubborn sibling less favorably. This practice should be avoided as it can harm the psychology and behavior of the "less-favored" child.

Parent's ignorance of proper methods of Raising children

Examples of this behavior include:

- The father rewards the child for using violence, perhaps by saying, "Take what is your right because you are a man."
- Parents excessively spoiling the child by fulfilling all his desires, leading him to expect instant gratification. When his desires are not met, this can lead to aggressive behavior.
- Both parents' resort to threats and physical punishment when dealing with their child at home.
- A societal tendency towards aggression, where a higher crime rate in society correlates with an

increased likelihood of the child becoming aggressive.

Ways of dealing with aggression

- Help the child understand that his behavior is not acceptable to others.
- Avoid hitting or yelling at the child and maintain appropriate boundaries.
- Recognize that punishment can have negative consequences; physical punishment may normalize violence, while verbal punishment can diminish the child's self-confidence, potentially leading to aggressive behavior.
- Teach the child about respecting the rights and possessions of others.
- Refrain from rewarding the aggressive child to avoid reinforcing the behavior and discouraging imitation from other children. Consider using "time outs" or ignoring the behavior while avoiding corporal or verbal punishment.
- Redirect the child's aggressive energy into constructive activities, with sports being an excellent option.
- Monitor the content your child consumes, including television shows, videos, DVDs, and computer games, as many may contain violent scenes or indirectly promote violence.
- Lead by example and avoid displaying marital or family conflicts in front of the child.

- Encourage empathy and perspective-taking by discussing how others may feel due to the child's actions.
- Teach conflict resolution skills like negotiation, compromise, and peaceful communication.
- Foster a supportive and nurturing environment at home where the child feels safe expressing emotions and seeking help when needed.
- Provide positive reinforcement for pro-social behaviors and acts of kindness towards others.
- Encourage social interactions and cooperative play with peers to develop empathy and teamwork skills.
- Set clear and consistent boundaries and logical consequences for breaking the rules.
- Practice active listening when the child expresses frustration or anger, validating their emotions while guiding them towards constructive responses.
- Offer opportunities for the child to practice self-regulation techniques, such as deep breathing, counting to ten, or taking a break when feeling overwhelmed.
- Seek professional guidance if the child's aggression persists or escalates despite intervention efforts.
- Collaborate with teachers, caregivers, and other adults involved in the child's life to consistently address aggressive behavior across different settings.

- Foster a culture of respect and understanding within the family, emphasizing tolerance, acceptance, and appreciation for diversity.
- Recognizing signs of illness and when to seek medical help

Stubbornness in children – causes and remedy

Parents must understand that stubbornness is common in all children, but its intensity and frequency can vary. Some degree of stubbornness is considered normal and shouldn't raise concerns. However, if stubbornness becomes a dominant aspect of a child's behavior, it can lead to more problematic behavior patterns.

Kinds of stubbornness in children

- Stubbornness coupled with rigid opinions and inflexible thinking, where the child insists on doing only what they want, regardless of correctness or logical reasoning.
- Stubbornness leading to neglect of important tasks like personal hygiene, refusal to follow adult instructions or requests, and resistance to adhering to set routines such as sleeping at specific times.

Causes of stubbornness in children

- Constantly denying the child's desires may provoke a desire for retaliation, manifested through stubbornness.
- Parents often misinterpret stubborn behavior as a sign of strong character in the child, inadvertently reinforcing it.
- Discord within the parental relationship can create a tense environment for the child, potentially contributing to stubbornness.
- Imposing rigid expectations regarding eating habits, clothing choices, or social etiquette can provoke rebellion and stubbornness in the child.
- Overindulging the child can also lead to the development of stubborn behaviors.
- Inconsistent discipline or boundaries may confuse the child, leading to stubbornness as they test limits.
- Lack of positive reinforcement for cooperative behavior may inadvertently reinforce stubborn tendencies.
- Modeling stubborn behavior in adults within the child's environment can normalize and encourage similar behavior in the child.
- High-stress levels or instability in the child's environment can exacerbate feelings of defiance and stubbornness as coping mechanisms.

- Overemphasis on competition or comparison with siblings or peers can fuel a need to assert independence through stubborn behavior.

Dealing with stubbornness

- Instead of responding to the child's stubbornness with equal stubbornness, communicate openly and persuasively to address the behavior effectively.
- Acknowledge and fulfill reasonable requests from the child to foster cooperation and reciprocal respect.
- Choose to overlook minor stubbornness rather than engage in futile arguments with the child.
- Express praise and positive reinforcement when the child cooperate and complies with parental requests.
- Avoid employing ineffective parenting methods such as excessive indulgence or rigid enforcement of specific manners, attire, or dietary habits.
- Allow the child some leeway for expressing opposition, as long as it remains respectful and non-disruptive while modeling appropriate behavior for them to emulate.
- Encourage autonomy and decision-making within reasonable boundaries to cultivate a sense of independence and responsibility in the child.
- Provide clear and consistent expectations and consequences for behavior to establish a structured and supportive environment for the child to thrive.

- Seek professional guidance or support if dealing with persistent or challenging stubbornness in the child to develop effective strategies for managing the behavior.

Fear is a universal emotion experienced by all individuals, characterized by a profound sense of unease or apprehension in response to perceived or anticipated danger. Children may exhibit fear towards stimuli that adults might consider ordinary or innocuous; when fear is rational and corresponds to a genuine threat, it is considered a normal response.

However, when fear becomes irrational or disproportionate, it may signify an abnormal psychological condition known as a phobia. Phobias typically stem from underlying psychological disorders or heightened levels of anxiety and stress.

Types of fear in children

- Fear of strangers
- Fear of separation from the mother or caregiver
- Fear of animals, darkness, thunder, and lightning
- Fear of imaginary beings or situations
- Fears linked to specific events or experiences, such as parental arguments, where the fear becomes

associated with particular objects or circumstances, like a toy or solitude.

Causes of fear in children

- Experiencing a specific traumatic event, like witnessing a traffic accident, encountering a threatening animal, or facing the sudden death of a relative.
- Observing a parent's fear of certain animals, insects, or darkness leads the child to mimic those fears.
- Exposure to frequent arguments between the child's parents.
- Watching frightening television programs or movies.
- Physical vulnerability in the child makes them more prone to fear than stronger children.
- Persistent criticism from adults causes the child to lose self-esteem and confidence.
- Aggressive interactions with other children or adults create an atmosphere of fear and intimidation.
- Seeking attention from parents by displaying fear, hoping to receive more care and concern.
- Making jests with the child about unrealistic scenarios, like threatening to take away body parts, which may be taken seriously by the child, inducing fear.

- Parents use threats of punishment or physical discipline as a means of control.
- Some mothers resort to inappropriate scare tactics, like warning the child that they will be harmed by animals or strangers if they misbehave.

Dealing with fears in children

- Parents should foster feelings of security and confidence in their children, understanding their fears and helping to dispel them.
- Avoid resorting to physical punishment for any reason. Instead, use dialogue and visual aids like pictures or toys to gradually ease the child's fear, ensuring it's done sensitively and at the child's pace.
- Refrain from mocking the child's fears; offer reassurance and comfort to calm them.
- Set a positive example by not displaying fear in front of the child and maintaining a stable home environment to prevent the development of psychological issues.
- Avoid reinforcing the child's fear by over-attending to them when they're afraid. Instead, provide balanced support to help them manage their emotions.
- Encourage open communication about the child's fears and experiences to diminish their anxiety and prevent future fears.

- Avoid using scare tactics to coerce the child into certain behaviors, as this can instill negative associations and anxieties.
- Introduce storybooks that highlight bravery and courage in a positive light, without introducing frightening elements, to promote positive attitudes toward overcoming fear.
- If the child's fear persists and escalates into a phobia, seek professional help from a psychiatrist or psychologist to address the issue effectively.

Jealousy in children – causes and remedy

Jealousy is a common emotion in children, stemming from their natural instincts. However, it's crucial to distinguish between normal jealousy, which children may experience but typically attempt to conceal, and abnormal jealousy, characterized by excessive and potentially harmful behaviors towards others.

The most important manifestations of jealousy in children

- Seeking attention by reverting to behaviors like drinking milk from a bottle.
- Sleeping in the mother's bed or displaying aggression towards siblings.
- Bedwetting during the night.
- Clinging to the mother and preferring to stay in her lap.

Causes of jealousy in children

- The arrival of a new baby, particularly if the mother shifts attention away from the older child to care for the newborn.
- Making comparisons between siblings, such as praising one child's attributes or achievements while neglecting to do so for the other or comparing their academic performance.
- The younger child feels jealous of the older sibling who receives hand-me-downs, leading to feelings of inferiority.
- Parents using harsh disciplinary measures or negative language when addressing conflicts between siblings.
- Encouraging selfish behavior in children due to ineffective parenting and socialization methods.

Types of jealousy in children

Jealousy in children can manifest in various ways, including:

- Engaging in constant crying, meddling with the belongings of others, and damaging or breaking their siblings' toys.
- Some children display jealousy by refusing to eat food offered to them, even if they are hungry, which can worry and upset the mother, leading her to provide more care and attention to the child.

- Clinging to the mother persistently, regardless of her attempts to encourage independence, particularly when the child perceives that her attention is directed towards caring for a new baby.
- Resorting to criticism and insults towards anyone who opposes or challenges them as a way to assert dominance and cope with feelings of jealousy.

Dealing with jealousy in children

- Treat all children equally and avoid favoritism or differential treatment based on age, gender, or abilities.
- Refrain from comparing one child to another, even with good intentions of motivating or encouraging them.
- Foster a spirit of cooperation among children and recognize and reward those demonstrating cooperative behavior.
- Avoid making jokes or teasing the children, as this can undermine their confidence and self-esteem.
- Be mindful of not overly focusing on the needs of a newborn baby, especially in the presence of older siblings, to prevent feelings of neglect or jealousy.
- Ensure that the older child does not feel neglected or sidelined due to the attention required by the newborn, and reassure them of their importance and value within the family.
- Engage children in cooperative activities and games that promote teamwork and collaboration, such as

building projects or group tasks, and ensure that rewards for participation are fair and equitable among all involved.

Bedwetting – causes and remedy

Bedwetting, also known as enuresis or involuntary urination, is considered one of the most common disorders in children. Determining if a child has a bedwetting problem depends on their age and developmental stage:

- Most children can sleep through the night without diapers by the age of two or three. However, studies show that about 20% of children wet the bed until age four. By the age of five, approximately 17% of males and 13% of females still experience bedwetting.
- Bedwetting is typically recognized as a concern by the age of four. If a child continues to experience bedwetting beyond this age, it is advisable to consult a doctor to assess the underlying causes of the issue.

It's essential to note that bedwetting is not necessarily linked to the depth of a child's sleep. Even children who sleep deeply can awaken when their bladders signal they are full.

Therefore, bedwetting should be evaluated based on age and frequency rather than solely on sleep patterns.

Causes of bedwetting
Physical causes
Such as a bladder infection, small bladder size, anemia, and intestinal worms.
Psychological causes
These are the significant causes of bedwetting in children:

- Arrival of a new baby in the family: The child may regress due to feeling overshadowed by the new arrival, leading to behaviors aimed at attracting attention.
- Fear of the dark and nightmares: Anxiety and fear during sleep can contribute to bedwetting episodes.
- Lack of harmony between the parents: Ongoing conflict and fighting between parents can create a stressful environment for the child, potentially leading to bedwetting as a response to this tension.
- Harsh treatment from the parents: If the child perceives harsh or cruel treatment regarding the bedwetting issue, they may react by bedwetting as a form of defiance or retaliation.
- Fear induced by media exposure: Exposure to frightening content on television or other media sources can evoke feelings of tension and anxiety in children, potentially contributing to bedwetting incidents.

Prevention and cure

- Acknowledge and praise the child for dry nights, offering specific rewards or kind words as encouragement while avoiding showing disappointment if bedwetting occurs.
- Educate the child on recognizing the sensation of a full bladder by encouraging ample fluid intake during the day until they learn to identify this feeling.
- Foster a supportive and comforting atmosphere at home to help alleviate any stress or anxiety the child may feel.
- Communicate to siblings the importance of refraining from teasing or making fun of the child experiencing bedwetting.
- Refrain from using threats or punishment in response to bedwetting incidents, as they can exacerbate the issue.
- Emphasize that attention, care, love, and security are crucial to addressing bedwetting.
- Monitor the content the child is exposed to on television and electronic games, avoiding violent scenes or content that may agitate or distress them.
- Limit the child's fluid intake for a reasonable period before bedtime to reduce the likelihood of bedwetting.

- Consider waking the child to use the restroom at night, but do so in moderation to avoid disrupting their sleep patterns excessively.
- If bedwetting persists despite these efforts, seek medical advice to identify underlying causes and determine appropriate interventions.

Delay in speaking – causes and remedy.

Many parents eagerly anticipate their child's first words, followed by the development of full sentences. However, some children experience delayed speech, with some not uttering their first word until three or four. Several factors contribute to this delay:

- Hearing impairment is a primary cause, varying in severity and onset. Some children have impaired hearing from birth, while others lose hearing after acquiring language skills.
- Low cognitive ability hinders early speech development, particularly in children with intellectual disabilities, whose language acquisition is notably slow.
- Speech abnormalities like tongue or vocal cord issues can also impede speech development.
- Feelings of insecurity due to a lack of love and care may contribute to delayed speech.
- Children raised by caregivers, especially those who don't speak the child's native language correctly,

may experience delayed speech due to parental busyness and reliance on caregivers.

- Parents' busy work schedules may result in prolonged childcare outside the home.
- Bilingualism, particularly if the family's language isn't prevalent in the child's environment, can affect language acquisition, especially if the child interacts with others who speak a different language.
- Excessive shyness in the child may also contribute to delayed speech.

Prevention and cure

- Ensure the child's hearing is functioning properly.
- Speak clearly and use short, repetitive sentences when communicating with the child.
- Listen attentively to the child, allowing them to finish speaking even if their words are unclear, and try to understand their message.
- Engage with the child face-to-face lovingly and kindly, creating a positive atmosphere for communication.
- Avoid pressuring the child to speak, which may hinder their progress.
- Use vocabulary related to tangible objects or people in the child's environment.
- Give the child time to respond when asked a question, allowing them a moment to express themselves in sounds or gestures.

- Prioritize communication with your child and avoid distractions from other tasks.
- Facilitate peer interaction by arranging playtime with slightly older children who can serve as language models.
- Encourage social interaction by allowing the child to play with other children.
- If the child's speech delay persists into the second year, seek advice from a specialist doctor.
- Maintain a positive attitude and refrain from showing frustration or disappointment with the child's speech development, which may exacerbate the situation.

Stuttering – causes and remedy

Stuttering, a common speech issue among children aged two to four years, can persist and impact the child's and parents' psychological well-being.

Early intervention is crucial, and implementing a home program can help the child overcome this challenge.

Causes of stuttering

- Hearing issues can contribute to stuttering as a physical cause.
- Psychological factors like extreme shyness, fear, and introversion can also play a role.

- Harsh treatment from parents exacerbates stuttering rather than alleviating it.
- Pushing the child to speak before they are developmentally ready can contribute to stuttering.
- Marital conflicts and ongoing arguments between parents create tension for the child.
- Feelings of insecurity, fear of punishment, or difficulty accepting their environment can also lead to stuttering.

Prevention and cure

- Avoid displaying any distress or frustration regarding the child's stuttering, whether through verbal or non-verbal cues.
- Refrain from pressuring the child to correct their speech.
- Provide ample opportunities for the child to express themselves, ensuring attentive listening until they finish speaking.
- Support the stuttering child in speaking progressively in front of peers of varying ages, promoting the rebuilding of their self-assurance.
- Resist correcting the child's pronunciation or asking for repetitions, which could heighten their panic and bewilderment.
- While offering encouragement, consider downplaying the issue to prevent exacerbating the child's concerns.

- If the problem persists, seek guidance from a speech pathologist to identify the underlying cause and appropriate intervention.

Delay in walking

Several factors contribute to the age at which a child begins walking independently, including genetic predisposition and overall health. Typically, most healthy children start walking by the end of their first year, persisting until they master walking independently around the age of one and a half years. However, this milestone varies; some children may commence walking earlier, around nine months, while others may not take their first steps until after eighteen months.

Causes of that include the following:

- Overreliance on a baby walker can impede the development of independent walking skills. If there's a persistent delay in walking despite this, consulting a doctor is advisable.
- Lack of self-confidence and fear of failure after initial attempts may hinder a child's progress. Reassurance and physical support can help build confidence until the child feels comfortable standing and taking steps.
- Some children may delay walking because they feel safer crawling, perceiving it as a protective

measure. Encouragement from the mother to transition to walking while the child is already crawling can be beneficial.

- Constant carrying of the child without allowing opportunities to practice walking can contribute to delayed walking.
- Excessive consumption of high-calorie foods like rice pudding, corn starch, and sweets leading to obesity may delay walking due to the child's weight. Moderation in diet is essential to prevent obesity-related delays in walking.
- Uncomfortable or slippery new shoes can hinder walking attempts. It's advisable not to use shoes until the child has learned to walk comfortably.

When is a child regarded as late in walking?

It's important to distinguish between delays in walking and actual walking problems. Typically, a child is considered late in beginning to walk if they reach eighteen months of age without attempting to walk.

However, it's advisable to wait until the child reaches two years of age before concluding that there may be a significant delay in walking.

Causes of delay in walking in children

- A significant factor contributing to a child's delayed walking could be hereditary factors. Therefore, the doctor will likely inquire about any family history of walking difficulties among siblings, parents, or other relatives.

- Illnesses like meningitis, brain infections, or central nervous system disorders may impede a child's walking ability.
- Inadequate intake of essential nutrients such as vitamins and proteins can hinder normal development and delay walking milestones.
- Certain muscular conditions like Hoffman disease or early muscular atrophy can affect the child's muscle function, potentially delaying their ability to walk.

Is there a remedy for delay in walking?

You don't need to actively teach your child to walk because when they reach the appropriate age and their muscles, nerves, and confidence are prepared, they will naturally begin walking. However, if your child hasn't started walking by their second birthday, it's essential to consult a doctor for necessary evaluations and tests.

Can the baby walker assist my child in learning to walk?

Many mothers believe that using a walker helps children learn to walk early. However, it doesn't aid in walking; it may hinder learning. According to Doctor Spock, children naturally push their feet forward without considering balance. Walking demands various skills that a child might not yet possess. Eventually, the child will learn to walk through their efforts, so why introduce something new, especially if it's more challenging?

Additionally, walkers are generally not recommended because they can lead to accidents. They enable the child to move quickly, increasing the risk of falling, particularly downstairs. Therefore, I do not recommend them at all.

Bow leggedness

Bow leggedness in children is a common issue that often causes concern among parents. However, in most cases, it is not linked to any illness. The legs typically return to their normal position within two or three years.

Causes that may lead to bow-leggedness

Physiological causes

The position of the fetus in the mother's uterus, such as crossed legs, can contribute to bow leggedness in children.

Non-physiological causes

- Issues with the growth of the shinbone
- Vitamin D deficiency in the child's diet resulting in rickets
- Leg length discrepancy
- Bone or joint problems
- Fractured bone or dislocated joint
- Neglected osteomalacia (soft bones)
- Severe obesity

Remedies

- If the child's bowleggedness persists, it's important to consult a doctor who can differentiate between pathological and ordinary physiological bowleggedness.
- In the case of osteomalacia (soft bones), treatment typically involves administering calcium and vitamin D supplements to the child.
- Sunlight exposure for a specific duration, done safely to avoid harm, can aid in addressing the condition.
- If these interventions prove ineffective, surgical correction may be necessary to straighten the legs.

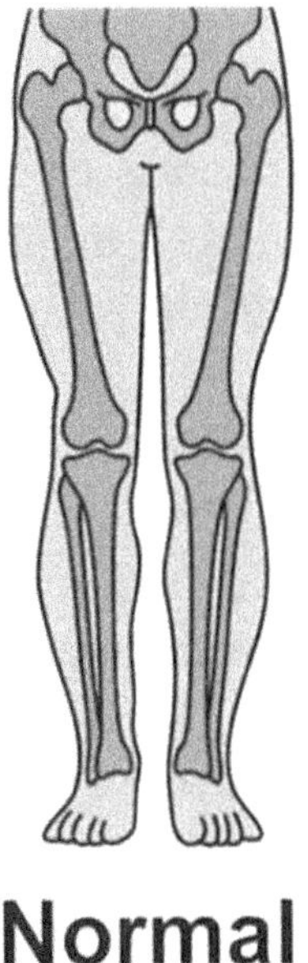

Normal

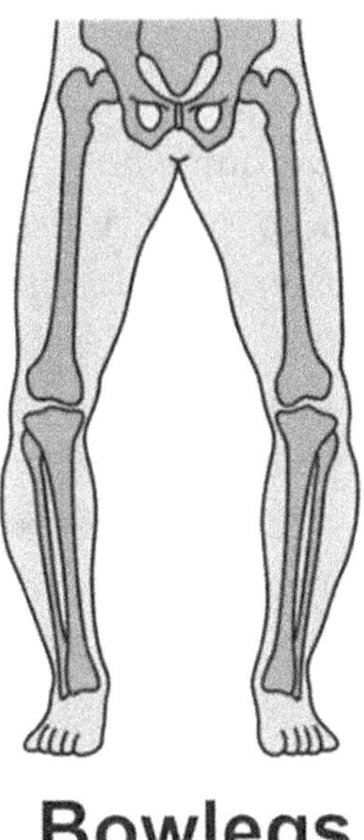

Bowlegs

Manners and etiquette

Etiquette and good manners are vital life skills that improve our whole character. Childhood is the ideal period to impart these life skills. A well-mannered youngster with decent manners will ultimately mature into a more self-assured adult.

This is a guide on proper behavior for children. We will cover everything, from etiquette at the table, being on time, and expressing appreciation to the fundamentals, like saying please and thank you. Continue reading to see them develop into the most honorable person you have ever desired!

It's never too late to begin instilling etiquette in your children. Parents must know the following list of thirty situation-specific good manners for children. Even though they may seem normal to you, they are crucial for helping your child develop social and emotional skills.

When living at home

Saying "Thank you" and "please"

This may be a fantastic place to start since it is one of the obvious entries in the list of good manners. "Thank You" fosters appreciation and thankfulness, whereas teaching your youngster to say "Please" fosters thoughtfulness. These kindness exercises help kids develop social skills and show more consideration and respect for the deeds of others.

Honoring both younger and older people

As they say, "Change starts at home," thus, if you want your kid to respect others outside of the house, you should start modeling such behavior at home first.

Seeking permission

Teaching kids to seek permission before touching or taking anything from someone else is important. It sends kids the message that permission is important, which you probably already know.

Refrain from Interrupting Talks

Free speech must be practiced, and "Let others finish before you speak" must be emphasized. Adopting this positive habit may greatly improve their communication skills in the workplace and classroom.

Lending a Helping Hand

Getting your child involved in domestic duties like sweeping, laundry, and room tidying up is a terrific approach to increase their helpful behavior.

Observing the Privacy of Others

To begin with, teach your child that every person on Earth needs their own time and space. It would benefit the learning process to knock on the door before entering the room, asking permission, not barging before attending the adult tea gatherings, etc.

When seated at the table

Putting away Smartphones

It has to be the most important table manners that young children may learn. Request they turn off all electronics for fifteen to twenty minutes at dinner.

With a Napkin

It is important to teach kids to always have a napkin on hand to prevent uncomfortable curry messes at the table.

Shutting Your Mouth When Eating

Children should take away from this an essential lesson: no one wants to know what's in their mouth, and they also certainly don't want to hear noises like chewing.

Asking before Leaving the Table

Asking for permission before leaving the table helps youngsters learn etiquette. It may be practiced when with people in a restaurant or at home.

When Visitors Are at Home

Letting Others in

Teach your youngster to open the door and welcome guests to the living room whenever they arrive at your house.

Grinning and shaking hands

Giving someone a solid handshake is a lovely way to meet them and makes them smile.

Stand Up When Elders Enter the Room

Children must learn the manners of standing and cheerfully welcoming the elderly and infirm as one aspect of demonstrating respect for them.

Taking Care of the Visitors

Teaching children to volunteer to serve visitors at home instills a sense of responsibility and courtesy.

Maintaining the Dialogue

Antisocial conduct and self-doubt stem from "Awkward Silences." Children must practice striking up and conversing with visitors at home. But it's important to properly teach them to walk the fine line between inconsequential bragging and threading discussions.

When You're the Visitor

Don't go uninvited

Teach the children to go only to their best friend's home when invited or for a special occasion.

Setting Stay Boundaries

It is important to teach children that they cannot spend as much time as they want at a friend's place. Instruct them to set a reasonable time limit when visiting someone's home.

Following the Host's House Rules

One who abides with the host's home rules is a good visitor. Youngsters must distinguish between adhering to the rules at home and the host's residence. Tell them to "do as the Romans do" while they are in Rome.

Providing Assistance
It is important to teach kids to appropriately support their hosts in their jobs rather than to burden them. It enables you to instill values of leadership, cooperation, and other critical social skills in your children.
Thanking Your Host for Their Hospitality
It falls under admiration and thanks in general. Expressing gratitude to the host family for their kindness and hospitality reinforces the importance of preserving ties among kids.

While You're on the Go
Refusing to Use Harsh Language
It is typical for kids to use derogatory language on the playground or at school. As a result, parents need to monitor and educate their kids on the negative effects of using vulgar language on other people.
Putting Sharing into Practice
Sharing, a crucial social skill, emphasizes the value of kindness and compassion, eventually advancing socioemotional growth. Children must be taught the value of sharing their food, possessions, and other material goods early.
Presenting Yourself to Other People
Children need to be taught how to introduce themselves to others; starting a discussion outside the house is a great approach. Starting with a kind smile, introducing yourself, asking for their name, and

stating, "Nice to meet you," is a great way to start the conventional hierarchy of introductions.

Reciprocating Customary Greetings

The younger generation has to learn how to politely return pleasantries when someone else makes the first approach. The typical responses to inquiries such as "How Are You?", "How Are You Doing?", "What's Going On?" Children need to be taught in, etc.

Acknowledging Your Mistakes

Children often believe that offering an apology—or offering one at all—makes them less worthy of respect. When such behavior persists until maturity, harmful features develop. Parents need to instill in their children the value of accepting responsibility for their deeds and offering an apology when necessary.

Saying "Excuse Me"

Children must be taught the manners of saying "Excuse Me" whenever necessary to instill compassion.

Not calling nicknames

Most students at school have a nickname for one another, but sometimes it may be harmful. It is crucial to take advantage of their sensitivity and advise them not to call their friends and relatives unpleasant names.

Following sportsmanship

It's inevitable to win and lose in life. Fostering in children a sense of sportsmanship entails training them to accept the accomplishments of others with dignity and modesty. This protects kids against unpleasant feelings like retaliation, resentment, and envy.

Avoiding Arguments with Others

It is best to prevent youngsters from getting into unnecessary arguments with people. It is best to promote teaching kids how to be patient, self-reliant, and peaceful to prevent them from becoming violent adults.

Maintaining Basic Hygiene

Teaching youngsters good manners—such as cleaning their hands, avoiding spitting on the street, tossing trash in the trash can, etc.—must continue until the behaviors become second nature. Children must be gently instructed to practice good hygiene at home and in public.

What Are the Advantages of Proper Behavior for Children?

The cornerstones of society are decency, civility, and etiquette. They are synonymous with displays of compassion and respect and contribute to developing positive relationships. Can you picture a world where everyone is uncivilized, violent, and unkind? You won't feel comfortable picturing it; we venture.

Therefore, it is impossible to overestimate the importance of manners to young children and preschoolers. Moreover, teaching children etiquette is crucial to creating a peaceful society.

Parents need to be aware of the following advantages of teaching their children manners:

Instills self-worth and confidence

A child's ability to behave appropriately in a certain circumstance or among a group of people highlights the confident streak ingrained in his nature. Teaching kids the fundamentals of social skills is a must for this. Etiquette and good manners are among them.

Fosters a feeling of Honor

Respect for oneself and other people is the foundation of good manners. A youngster ultimately understands appreciating individuals outside their family when they learn to respect themselves.

Encourages Bonding

A kid raised with manners and etiquette can benefit from having good relationships with their elders, classmates, cousins, and other family members. The foundation of life is human interactions. Teaching your children the value of their formative years will benefit them for the rest of their lives.

Enhances Interpersonal Skills

Children's academic and professional career development depends on their ability to communicate. Therefore, good manners and etiquette may help you improve relationships and communication abilities.

Brings Joy

A youngster experiences delight and profound satisfaction when they understand how their actions affect others around them favorably. Their happiness further opens up a world of favorable opportunities.

What Can Parents Do to Help Their Children Learn Manners?

Every parent aims to raise a kid who exhibits manners and other basic decency. However, the majority of parents are unaware of how much they influence their kids' personalities. The automobile starts to slide at that point. If you believe that you fit that description, don't give up. "Better late than never," they say.

Below is a list of little details to remember while you continue teaching your children politeness.

Exemplary Conduct

This is the best technique to instill manners and etiquette in your children. As parents, we must model positive traits for our children. Becoming kind to them is the first step in becoming an example for them. The greatest approach is to speak to your children in a calm manner that you would want them to exhibit. Show your child proper manners by modeling them with your behaviors, and see how fast they pick them up and apply them.

Commencing with the Early Lessons

The greatest time to begin teaching your child manners and etiquette is as soon as they become one year old. Are you wondering why at such an early age? By this age, newborns usually start to watch and try to imitate their parents' behavior. You may teach your baby politeness, for instance, by placing their toys in the toy basket. After a few days of repetition, observe how eagerly the baby grows up to repeat the behavior. Similarly, teach your children manners early on—don't wait until they start preschool—by teaching them phrases like "please" and "thank you."

Give Examples

Although rules establish etiquette and manners, they may also be reinforced by examples to eventually become habits. As a parent, you are responsible for outlining particular situations and talking with your child about what has to be done and when. Children must respond appropriately and comprehend the nature of the situation. Therefore, the next time you teach children etiquette, have some activity cards or placards available to help prepare them for appropriate responses, actions, behavior, and speech.

Maintain Consistency

The results of teaching good manners take time to attain, just like any other learning. You must repeat the behaviors and establish clear expectations if you want your youngster to continuously exhibit appropriate manners and etiquette. For instance, ensure your youngster does away with his phone at the dinner table until it becomes second nature. If your youngster forgets to stand when adults enter the room, intervene to remind them. A child receives more effective tutoring when their parents are more consistent in modeling kindergarten etiquette.

Accurately and politely

Parents often discipline their children when they disobey their instructions to be as consistent as possible. This is a serious warning sign that will do more damage than good. Determine what went wrong with your original teaching strategy if your youngster struggles to learn the material. Make it normal for your child to try harder than other kids to behave politely at all times. When you gently reprimand someone, they will see that you appreciate them and try to do better the next time.

Congratulate Excellent Conduct

Children are no different from adults in that they may feel great pleasure from little acts of gratitude and compliments. Parents are responsible for encouraging their children's efforts and giving them a sense of worth. For instance, praise them when they appropriately say "thank you." Alternatively, express your pride in your child when they assist without you having to remind them. Acknowledging these little victories in life teaches individuals that being courteous makes others happy and reinforces good behavior.

Teaching aids have evolved to become more innovative and easily available. The engaging activities listed below may help parents better teach manners and etiquette in the comfort of their own homes.

Good Manners chart

This is accomplished using several downloadable good manners charts found online. They provide a list of kid-friendly good manners that are situation-specific. Allow your youngster to take the lead by putting them in the kitchen or on the refrigerator.

"I Caught You Being Good" jar

Put a label on an old jar and write, "I Caught You Being Good." Record it on paper and place it inside the jar every time your youngster behaves well and shows manners. Every month, count the number of chits in the jar and give your youngster a prize for doing so.

Good Manners journal

Keeping a notebook is an excellent method to monitor your child's etiquette. Urge your child to jot down at least ten manners he uses regularly at school. Reward the number of well-mannered behaviors on the list and the recipient's age.

Tabletop Games

Children learn important life skills more effectively when a fun component is included in the lesson.

The board game "Mind Your Manners" is one example that may work. It's readily accessible both online and at nearby shops.

The Ribbon and the Beads

You may use this game to see whether your youngster shows thankfulness in return. Take a package of beads and a ribbon in your child's favorite color. Every time your youngster expresses appreciation or says "thank you," add a bead to the ribbon. And tie a knot every time she fails to express appreciation. By the end of the month, count the beads and give them a prize based on your established limit.

Reading a Book About Manners

It's time to read a book to your children to instill excellent manners. To complete this task, utilize the top children's reading websites. Since the beginning of time, stories have surely had a significant influence on the characters of children. Parents may choose the alternatives that appeal to them from various available possibilities. Please Say Please, Dude, That's Rude-Get Some Manners, Are you Quite Polite, Perfect Pigs: An Introduction to Manners, and A is for Attitude: An Alphabet For Living are a few books on manners that are highly recommended.

Let's Bring Up Well-Behaved Children!

We observed that educating kids about etiquette has a lot of advantages. We need to raise kinder, more loving, and more compassionate children if we want society to remain polite and orderly. Although it may seem impossible to teach etiquette to young children, it is possible to do so by making little but meaningful changes in day-to-day activities.

Parents need to shape themselves and their children so that basic manners become second nature. Okay, so what's the rule? You will harvest what you sow. The best present parents can offer their kids is the gift of manners and politeness.

Answers to Common Questions (FAQs)

What makes manners different from etiquette?
While etiquette refers to a set of guidelines or behavior, manners generally refer to the generalized behavior that conveys an individual's attitude. While turning off the phone in a movie theater, sitting up straight at the dinner table, and other behaviors are instances of excellent manners, respecting elders, speaking courteously, and being nice are examples of etiquette. Since both are essential to society's operation, polite people are likelier to observe manners correctly.

Is it too late to start teaching my second-grader proper manners?
Not at all. Parents need to keep in mind that politeness cannot be imposed. Instead, they may be absorbed via practice and observation at home. Second, the secret to children's good manners is consistent communication between parents and children. The children have faith in you when you have faith in yourself. The finest resources for kids between the ages of five and seven

are motivational speeches and novels with deep content.

Do polite behavior and a prosperous future life go hand in hand?

When a youngster learns appropriate manners, he repeats them until they are ingrained in him. Children who behave well greatly influence others, increasing their confidence and sense of self-worth. Success is inevitable when a youngster develops into a graceful, self-assured, kind, and caring adult.

Prayers

For a youngster, prayer is an integral part of their lives. It facilitates their ability to concentrate on what matters and forge deep connections with God. However, if you are unfamiliar with any prayers, it may be challenging to teach them to youngsters.

You may educate your children about God and the art of prayer by using any of the numerous kid-friendly prayers available. These nine are our top picks:

Every Day Prayer

Your youngster may recite this brief, easy prayer each day. It demonstrates to them how to begin their prayers each day and aids in helping them concentrate on what matters:

He wakes me up; He makes me sleep.
Provides for me the food I eat.
When I cry, I call on Him,
Because I know with Him, I win.
Even though the hardest day,
I trust in Him in every way.
He's the One who sees me through,
Jesus lives; I know it's true.
With loving kindness, He smiles at me.
Because He died, I am free.
Lord, for all, I thank you so,
I know you'll never let me go!
– Esther Lawson

The Serenity Prayer

Children may employ the well-known Serenity Prayer to help them cope with difficult circumstances. It reminds people that even under trying circumstances, they may depend on God for support and direction:

God, grant me the serenity to accept the things I cannot change,
Courage to change the things I can,
And wisdom to know the difference.
– Reinhold Niebuhr

The Lord's Prayer

This one is possibly one of the most well-known prayers for adults and children. It is a powerful prayer that addresses a wide range of significant life issues, from pleading with God for direction and protection to expressing gratitude for all of his blessings:

Our Father in Heaven,
hallowed be thy name,
Thy kingdom come,
Thy will be done,
On earth as in heaven.
Give us today our daily bread.
Forgive us our sins,
As we forgive those, who sin against us.
Lead us not into temptation,
But deliver us from evil.
For the kingdom, the power, and the glory are yours
now and forever.
Amen.

– Matthew 6:9-13

The Lord is My Light
This prayer is a lovely approach to help your kid, particularly in times of fear or uncertainty, express their faith and confidence in God. It serves as a reminder that God is constantly there to keep an eye on and defend them:

Lord, I know you're my light;
My path shines brightly through the night.
I know that your love comes true,

and prayers that I say come straight from you.
I know you're my shield in battle;
My sword and my armor when danger rattles.
And though no one's watching me now,
Your eyes are always focused on me somehow.
Your love is so strong, Lord, like the mountains that
soar,
And I know that your prayers are always right at my
door.
– Lindsey Burgess

The Lord Is My Rock and Guide
Children are urged by this prayer to put their trust in
God for guidance in life. It serves as a reminder that
people may rely on Him for guidance throughout trying
times and that He will see them through:
Lord, You are my Rock and Guide;
You lead me through life's dark tide.
Your love is true, Your will is right,
And You protect me day and night.
I know that when I am lost,
You'll help me find the path again.
In times of trouble and distress,
You grant Your peace within my heart.
– Ruth Ann Mahaffey

Thank You, God, for My Family
This is a brief children's prayer. It's ideal for saying a prayer before a meal or taking a moment to thank your loved ones:

Thank you, God, for the world so sweet
Thank you, God, for the food we eat
Thank you, God, for the birds that sing
Thank you, God, for everything
Amen.

– E. Rutter Leatham

Prayer for Protection
Children may remain secure and protected throughout their everyday lives by using the potent prayer for protection. It serves as a crucial reminder to put their faith in God, who will always be there to protect and lead them:

Dear God,
I know that You are my protector.
You watch over me each day.
Please keep me safe from harm.
I know that You are always with me,
And I trust in Your care. Amen.

– Unknown

Prayer for Mealtime Blessings
A lovely way to show thanks for the meal you and your family are going to consume is with this little prayer.

Saying this before meals or whenever you want to express gratitude for your blessings is ideal:

Bless us, O Lord,
And these thy gifts
Which we are about to receive.
Through Christ, our Lord. Amen.

– Unknown

Bedtime Prayer

A prayer before bedtime is a wonderful way to close out the day and express gratitude for all that God has blessed us with. It serves as a reassuring reminder that God is always keeping an eye on us and will defend us at night:

Here I lay me down to sleep
To thee, O Lord, I give my soul to keep,
Wake I ever, Or, Wake I never;
To thee, O Lord, I give my Soul to keep forever.

– George Wheler

Why Offer Up Prayers?

To communicate with God, use prayer. It is a means of getting in touch with God. By praying, you allow a higher power than yourself to guide and assist you. Praying for anything is a great way for kids to express gratitude to God for His benefits or to ask for assistance with difficulty.

Children may learn about God and develop a meaningful relationship via praying. They may come to know who He is and how they can depend on Him for help throughout their lives by praying.

Let's offer prayers!

Frequently Asked Questions

When is the ideal time for kids to begin praying?

Given the uniqueness of each kid, there is no universal response to this question. While some kids may not be interested in prayer until they are older, others could be prepared to begin praying very early. When a youngster is ready to begin praying, it is ultimately up to the parents to choose.

How can I support my kid in praying?

You may assist your youngster in praying in a few ways:

- Urge them to share their thoughts with God, including anything for which they are thankful or about which they are anxious.
- Instruct children to keep God in mind at all times and assist them in creating a prayer pattern that includes saying prayers before bed or during meals.
- Regular scripture reading and prayer can help your kid develop a connection with God.

How might prayer help my kid grow spiritually?

A child's spiritual growth cannot be completed without prayer since it fosters a closer relationship with God and a more profound comprehension of their religion. Children may get wisdom, consolation, and tranquility from God via prayer. Prayers for children may also contribute to the family's general well-being by fostering a culture of love and collaboration.

Toilet training

Toilet training should commence when the child recognizes the urge to urinate, and the mother should guide the child through the process patiently, avoiding coercion.

How can I determine if my child is ready for toilet training?

- The child displays discomfort when their diaper is dirty.
- They can maintain dryness for at least two hours.
- They comprehend basic commands like "Go," "Come," or "Give me."
- They can independently dress and undress without assistance.
- Physical signs, such as tugging at clothes, sitting, squatting, or verbal cues, indicate their need to urinate.

- The child can sit and walk unaided.
- They desire to please their parents and participate positively.

What is the right age for my child to start using the toilet?

Commencing toilet training isn't bound by a specific age for every child. Instead, it's based on assessing your child's physical abilities and cognitive readiness. Normally, this readiness emerges between 18 and 24 months, although some children may not exhibit the necessary skills until they reach 3 or 4 years old.

A step-by-step guide to toilet training

Step 1

Purchase the essentials for toilet training. One of the primary items to acquire is a potty, a vital tool in teaching your child how to use the toilet. Additionally, consider obtaining small rewards to incentivize your child each time they successfully use the potty. Picture books or DVDs can also be valuable resources for your child to learn about toilet usage.

Step 2

Educate your child to communicate with you when they feel the urge to urinate, but be patient as this skill may take time to develop. Initially, your child may indicate the need to urinate after the fact rather than beforehand. In such instances, refrain from scolding or frightening them. Remember that this process may require time and consistency, and success may vary from one attempt to another.

Step 3

Educate your child about the names of body parts and terms for urine and feces to ensure they understand your instructions when teaching them toilet use.

This foundational knowledge will aid in effective communication during the training process.

Step 4

Familiarize your child with sitting on the potty by encouraging them, even when they don't want to urinate. This helps them become accustomed to the potty. However, refrain from forcing them to sit on it, as children at this age tend to resist instructions. Avoid pressuring or coercing them into using the potty.

Step 5

Once your child is comfortable sitting on the potty and can express their need to urinate, explain to them that when they sit on the potty, they need to lift up their clothes. Pay attention to any signs or gestures indicating that they need to urinate. When you notice these signs, guide them to the potty and help them sit on it. If your child defecates in their diaper before reaching the potty, guide them to the potty again. Afterward, remove their diaper and transfer the feces into the potty, reinforcing the connection between sitting on the potty and defecating.

Step 6

Transitioning from the potty to the toilet is a natural progression once your child is comfortable using the potty and understands the sensation of needing to urinate. Encourage your child to use the potty and the toilet simultaneously for a short period.

If your child resists using the toilet, continue to offer both options until they recognize the toilet as the appropriate place to relieve themselves. This dual approach can help ease the transition from the potty to the toilet.

Step 7

Nighttime training should commence once your child can stay dry and clean throughout the day but still struggles to remain dry overnight due to their body not being mature enough to sense the need to urinate while asleep.

To assist your child in staying dry at night, avoid giving them large amounts of liquids before bedtime. Keep the potty near their bed and encourage them to call for you if they wake up at night so you can bring it to them.

Note

Toilet training requires considerable patience, so it's important not to expect rapid results. Avoid rebuking or punishing your child for any mistakes or if they show reluctance to start training.

Instead, encourage your child to cooperate and respond positively to the training process. Remember to reward your child when they progress or show effort in learning to use the toilet. Positive reinforcement and patience are key to successful toilet training.

Children and television

Television can sometimes feel like a convenient babysitter for parents, but excessive TV time can harm children's development. While I don't advocate for a complete ban on TV, it's essential to set limits and choose programs wisely. Here are some guidelines:

- Limit TV time to one or two hours per day.
- Select programs based on educational content and principles.
- Encourage discussion between parent and child about what they watch to enhance understanding and critical thinking skills.

Negative effects of watching television

The consequences of excessive television watching on children are significant and diverse:

- TV time replaces natural activities crucial for brain development and talent nurturing, such as interacting with parents and engaging in mentally stimulating games, leading to decreased physical and social activities.
- Prolonged TV viewing is linked to childhood obesity due to sedentary behavior and unhealthy eating habits while watching.
- It distracts children from academic studies and social interactions.
- Studies indicate that every hour spent watching TV leads to a 10% decrease in alertness and focus, aversion to reading, and reduced critical thinking.
- Television negatively affects mental and psychological well-being, diminishing innovative thinking, weakening social skills, and fostering apathy.
- Exposure to violent content on TV can induce fear, nightmares, and violent behavior in children.
- There's a risk of children encountering indecent or pornographic material on television, especially when families watch together without considering the content's suitability for children.
- Advertisement exposure, particularly for unhealthy food products, influences children's food

preferences and contributes to unhealthy eating habits, potentially leading to obesity.

Advice to help turn the television from Being a destructive force to bring something beneficial to children

To mitigate the negative effects of television on young children, here are some guidelines to follow:

- Children under two years old should avoid television altogether.
- Avoid using TV as a babysitter; watch programs with your children and discuss them to help them distinguish between reality and fiction.
- Limit your child's TV time to one or two hours per day, based on agreed-upon shows.
- Lead by example and limit your own TV consumption.
- Encourage alternative activities like sports, hobbies, and physical play.
- Avoid eating meals while watching TV.
- Familiarize yourself with the content of the programs before allowing your child to watch.
- Choose cartoons without violent or aggressive scenes, avoiding shows that promote negative behaviors.
- Prioritize homework and chores before TV time.
- Keep control of the remote to regulate viewing habits effectively.

Smoking

When a mother smokes, the harmful chemicals, especially nicotine, in cigarette smoke affect breast milk, weakening the child's immunity and making them susceptible to lung disease, slow growth, and heart problems. Apart from the risks of diseases, there's the issue of setting a poor example. Every smoking parent should ask themselves: "Am I being a good role model for my child?" The answer is undoubtedly no, as no mother wants her child to smoke. Smoking in front of a child is essentially teaching them, and when they become old enough to smoke, they won't hesitate. Therefore, both parents need to quit smoking, motivated by their love for their child, to break the habit.

Arguments between the parents in front of the children

There's a distinction between constructive discussions, where parents calmly express differing viewpoints to resolve issues, and heated arguments filled with conflict in front of children, potentially escalating to hurtful language and insults, deeply affecting the children's psyche.

For young children, stability is crucial; they need to feel safe and secure and develop confidence in themselves and those around them, which is unlikely in a household rife with parental conflict.

Research indicates that children raised in such environments are more likely to argue with peers, making argumentativeness a recurring pattern.

Furthermore, these arguments deprive children of positive role models, eroding their trust and respect for their arguing parents. This lack of guidance can hinder the child's success and stability, potentially leading to resentment towards one or both parents and a disconnection from the family.

Parents must reflect on whether such an environment can nurture successful and psychologically stable children. Dr. Fifaan Ahmad Fu'ad, a Psychiatry Professor at Helwan University, emphasizes the detrimental impact of tense marital relationships on a child's character.

It instills fear and insecurity, weakening academic performance and concentration due to heightened stress levels. As children witness parental conflicts, their own mental and emotional well-being suffers, affecting their ability to learn and engage effectively in school.

The solution to all of that is as follows:

- Parents should serve as role models for their children and educate them on expressing their thoughts calmly and logically, ensuring they respect others' rights.
- It's crucial to select appropriate times and settings to address issues, avoid discussions when the family is tired, and during meals or bedtime to prevent negative effects on the children.
- Parents must acknowledge that ongoing marital disputes can eventually lead to psychological and physical issues for children, notably nightmares and bedwetting.
- To alleviate daily stresses experienced by family members, consider taking trips or bringing children along to visit loved ones, like grandparents.
- Above all, parents should recognize their pivotal role as influencers in their children's lives, understanding that they profoundly shape their children's attitudes and behaviors.

Hitting children

Children rely on their parents for protection, security, and love. When parents resort to hitting and violence as the primary means of discipline, it can lead to frustration and confusion in the child as they experience violence from those expected to provide safety and security.

Physical punishment creates individuals who fear any confrontation and are hesitant to take action, even when beneficial, for fear of physical harm. Additionally, the child's personality may become introverted and unable to cope with pain.

Exposure to parental hitting and violence can result in the child becoming violent and stubborn, often resorting to arguments and aggression with siblings and peers.

While some social psychology experts advocate for smacking as a disciplinary measure, it must be understood that this does not involve severe physical or psychological harm. Children may be smacked for discipline, provided it does not lead to psychological complexes or increased stubbornness.

However, many psychologists and educators argue against smacking as a punishment for children, preferring rational disciplinary methods that avoid physical and psychological harm, which can undermine the child's dignity. They advocate for alternative approaches that prioritize the well-being and development of children without resorting to violence.

Things that can reduce smacking of children

- Take some time to unwind and relax. Many parents resort to hitting their children when they are overwhelmed and unable to find time for themselves.
- Offering your child alternatives is preferable to resorting to smacking. For instance, if your child is playing with food, it's better to warn them of consequences like, "Either stop playing with your food or face a punishment."
- When your child accidentally breaks something at home, avoid hitting them. Reacting with violence will only breed anger and a desire for revenge in the child. Instead, encourage accountability by making them responsible for repairing or replacing the item, perhaps by deducting the cost from their pocket money. Emphasize the importance of taking responsibility for one's actions.
- Discipline the child by depriving them of privileges they enjoy, such as restricting computer usage, withholding pocket money, or canceling planned trips. These methods are more effective than resorting to physical punishment.

Insulting or swearing at children

Many parents opt for verbal punishment to correct their children's misbehavior, believing it to be a better alternative to physical punishment.

However, recent research and scientific studies indicate otherwise, highlighting that verbal rebukes can be equally damaging to a child's psyche.

Insulting children can harm their self-respect and self-confidence, as it instills a sense of worthlessness in them. When children are consistently subjected to rebukes and insults for their mistakes, they may internalize inappropriate language and develop a sharp tongue in their interactions with family members.

According to Dr. Sayyid Subhi, a professor of mental health, any form of punishment undermines a child's self-respect, as it conveys the message that they are insignificant.

In conclusion, mothers must treat their young children with respect, fostering an environment where they feel valued and develop confidence in themselves and those around them. Moreover, when communicating with children, it's important to carefully choose words that reflect the behavior and language you wish to cultivate in them.

Encouraging Play and Learning

Play can be defined as "an activity or a series of activities for entertainment or fun," as described by 'Adnaan 'Aarif Muslih in 1999. It involves independent movement or activity to bring pleasure or enjoyment, typically requiring both mental energy and physical movement.

Types of play

Various types of play can be classified into different categories:

Based on the number of participants:

- Playing alone
- Playing in a group

Based on the structure of the play:

- Spontaneous play without rules
- Play governed by rules (games)

Based on the type of play:

- Boisterous play
- Quiet play
- Play that promotes coordination of movements and muscle growth
- Play that is primarily cognitive, involving thinking and reasoning skills

Benefits of play

The play offers numerous benefits to children, including:

- Release of physical and mental tension.
- Expression and discharge of suppressed feelings, aggressive tendencies, and negative emotions through toy interaction.
- Opportunity for learning and developing potential, such as acquiring new skills and overcoming challenges.
- Evidence of functioning imagination, as children engage in symbolic play where everyday objects take on new roles and meanings.
- Enrichment of the child's life with various activities.
- Increase the child's knowledge of the environment and understanding of the world.
- Opportunity for expressing needs that may be difficult to articulate in real life.
- Utilization of senses and reasoning, enhancing cognitive development.
- Facilitate social interaction and integration with others.
- Fulfilling the fundamental need for change, preventing boredom, and promoting adaptability.

Things to bear in mind when selecting toys

When selecting toys for children, it's important to consider the following factors:

- Align the toy with the child's interests and preferences.
- Ensure it's suitable for the child's age and stage of development.
- Select toys that promote learning and emotional and social growth.
- opt for versatile toys that offer various play options.
- Check for harmful chemicals that could jeopardize the child's health.
- Choose attractive, user-friendly, and reasonably priced toys.
- Prioritize toys with appealing colors, lightweight design, smooth texture, and easy-to-clean features.
- Ensure safety by selecting toys that are not small enough to be swallowed and lack sharp corners or metal parts.
- Seek toys that provide both short-term and long-term entertainment and can be utilized in multiple ways to keep the child engaged and happy. Toys that offer options for disassembly and reassembly or are versatile in usage are particularly enjoyable.

Developing the child's skills through play
Make-believe and expressive games

- Symbolic play enables children to manage their emotions by expressing anger, sadness, and anxiety, allowing them to vocalize their thoughts on positive and negative experiences.
- Role-playing games facilitate understanding different perspectives as children embody roles such as father, doctor, or teacher.
- Make-believe activities foster innovative thinking and creativity in children.
- Through these imaginative games, children acquire social skills, including cooperation, active listening, role assignment, and problem-solving.
- Engaging in pretend play aids children in comprehending the roles they enact, helping them overcome fears or uncertainties associated with those roles; for instance, assuming the role of a doctor may alleviate apprehensions about medical visits.
- Symbolic play contributes to developing motor control and hand-eye coordination in children.

Roles that the child can play

In make-believe play, children can assume various roles, including those of fathers, mothers, teachers, doctors, elderly individuals, and more.

Artistic play

Artistic play provides children the opportunity and tools to express themselves creatively, positively channeling their energy and nurturing their appreciation for artwork. Through this type of play, children utilize various raw materials like modeling clay, scissors, and colored pens, which aid in developing fine motor skills and hand control, essential for later learning how to write. Additionally, artistic play enhances hand-eye coordination and enables children to explore the characteristics of the materials they interact with.

Engaging in artistic play also fosters a sense of achievement and boosts self-confidence in children, particularly when they create artwork and receive support, affection, and praise from their parents. Displaying their creations in a special place in the house further reinforces their sense of accomplishment and pride.

Constructive play

This type of quiet, individual play allows children to cultivate a rich imagination while exercising their muscles through movement, contraction, and expansion. Constructive play comes in various forms, and investing in toys like blocks, Lego, and similar items is highly beneficial for children. Here are some advantages of constructive play:

- Constructive play is closely linked to various stages of a child's physical and mental development. Initially, it involves placing objects next to each other. As the child progresses intellectually, they will attempt to stack them on top of each other to form structures like pyramids or walls.
- Children derive happiness from being able to construct shapes with the materials they are playing with.
- This type of play teaches children skills that contribute to the development of scientific thinking, such as comparing, predicting, observing, analyzing, understanding balance, and recognizing differences and similarities between shapes.
- Constructive play introduces children to basic mathematical concepts such as classification, sequencing, understanding area, and counting.
- Engaging in constructive play enhances a child's planning ability. As they progress, they transition from random construction to planning what they want to build, fostering their planning abilities.

Cognitive play

This type of play involves activities requiring the child to concentrate and think critically to achieve a goal. It assesses the child's ability to solve problems and figure things out. Cognitive play includes puzzles of varying difficulty, memory games, matching games, sorting games, and various language-based activities such as describing, explaining, and distinguishing by sound.

Cognitive play is crucial for developing the child's mental abilities, expanding their understanding, and fostering their thinking ability. It enhances problem-solving skills, contributes to developing linguistic abilities, and helps the child to analyze, focus, and innovate. Additionally, cognitive games aid in the development of hand-eye coordination.

Active play

Dr. Jihan al-Qaadi, the head of the Egyptian Learning Difficulties Society, emphasizes the importance of play during this stage, focusing on muscle development, coordination, and overall mobility. Outdoor play, particularly in parks, is beneficial as it exposes the child to sunlight, which aids in treating conditions like bow-leggedness. Active play brings joy and adventure into the child's life and contributes to their physical well-being.

Parents should select toys that promote these activities, such as cars and animals on wheels, small trunks or bikes, and balls for throwing and kicking. Engaging in play with their children, whether in public parks or social clubs, allows parents to encourage these active behaviors.

As children reach their third year, parents should consider introducing them to sporting activities suitable for their age.

Early childhood toys should focus on developing large muscles by swinging, jumping, balancing, and biking.

Active play also fosters social skills, teaching children the importance of cooperation, sharing, team spirit, and responsibility. Games like hide-and-seek, jumping games, and ball throwing and catching help children learn these values and introduce them to positive competition, motivating them to progress and succeed in a group setting.

Examples of fun and educational games for children

Games that the child can play in the first year of life

Note:

More important than constantly training your child to acquire these skills is giving him hugs and showing him love when he succeeds in playing any of these games. This emotional support and affection are vital for fostering a sense of security, confidence, and emotional well-being in the child.

Problem-solving game

Teach your child problem-solving skills by engaging them in activities like placing a cornflake or piece of dry bread in the opening of a small-necked bottle and letting them figure out how to retrieve it, such as by turning the bottle upside down. Similarly, toys like stacking rings can help them develop these skills as they figure out how to arrange the rings on a cylinder base. These activities encourage cognitive development and problem-solving abilities in children.

Eating with a spoon

Teaching your child to eat with a spoon can be a playful activity. Start by giving them spoons to play with, observing as they explore, and sometimes dropping them. As they show interest, place a small piece of banana on a spoon and guide it into their mouth, gradually introducing different foods. Soon enough, they'll learn to mimic eating with a spoon by placing it on an empty plate and feeding themselves. This playful approach helps them develop important social and motor skills.

Suspended toys or mobiles

You can enhance your baby's crib area by hanging toys above it, either with ready-made options or by creating your own. Simply purchase some string and attach fabric dolls or toys to it, then hang it within the baby's view. This simple addition can provide entertainment and stimulation for your little one.

"Musical gloves"

Introducing your baby to sound localization can be done by engaging with gloves equipped with small bells. Encourage your baby to shake the gloves in different locations until they notice the sound and associate it with the movement of the gloves. This interactive game fosters the development of auditory skills and spatial awareness in your child.

Bathtub toys

Bath time can also be playtime for your baby! Enhance the experience by adding toys like boats, rubber ducks, or colorful plastic fruits such as lemons, oranges, and apples to the bathtub. These toys make bath time more enjoyable and stimulate your baby's sensory exploration and hand-eye coordination.

Peek-a-boo

Playing peek-a-boo with your child is fun and helps them understand object permanence, the concept that things continue to exist even when they can't be seen. Sit near your child and cover your face with your hands or a cushion, then ask, "Where did Mama go?" before revealing your face and saying, "Here I am!" You can make the game more exciting by hiding behind furniture or doors and surprising your child when you pop out. This game teaches your child that you will always come back, even if you briefly disappear.

Walking games

Playing games with your toddler as they learn to walk can be fun and beneficial for their development. Encourage flexibility and coordination by helping them walk in different directions—sideways, backward, and forwards. You can trot like a horse or walk on tiptoes to prompt imitation. Stretch your arms forward while walking or vary your pace between quick and slow, and invite them to follow your lead. These activities engage them physically and help strengthen their motor skills and balance.

Building games

Playing with blocks of various shapes, sizes, and colors is enjoyable and beneficial for your child's development. However, ensure that the blocks are not too small to avoid any risk of swallowing. Building sets made of wood or plastic with large pieces are also great options as they encourage creativity and invention. These activities foster cognitive, spatial awareness, and fine motor skills as your child explores different ways to construct and create with the blocks.

Shape sorting games

Toys like boards or boxes with openings of various shapes and corresponding blocks are excellent for helping children learn about shapes and develop their problem-solving skills. These toys encourage tactile exploration as children manipulate the blocks to fit them into the corresponding holes. Additionally, they promote cognitive development by teaching children to recognize and match shapes, fostering spatial reasoning and hand-eye coordination.

Dominoes

Playing dominoes with colorful and pictorial pieces is a great way for children to engage socially while developing their cognitive and matching skills. Children practice observation, critical thinking, and pattern recognition by searching for matches between the pictures, shapes, or colors on the domino pieces. Additionally, playing games like dominoes with others helps children learn important social skills such as taking turns, following rules, and good sportsmanship.

Telling colors apart

Playing color identification games like this is a fantastic way to engage a child's cognitive skills and enhance their vocabulary. By asking the child to identify objects based on color, you're helping them develop their color recognition abilities while reinforcing their understanding of different objects and their names. It's a simple yet effective way to encourage learning through play and interaction.

Games to develop the sense of hearing

Using everyday objects to teach a child about different sounds is a great way to engage their auditory senses and expand their understanding of the world around them. By associating specific objects with distinct sounds, you're helping them develop their auditory discrimination skills and enriching their vocabulary and cognitive abilities. Plus, it's a fun and interactive way to learn together!

Acting games

Encouraging a child to imitate positive role models through play is a wonderful way to foster their imagination and social skills. By engaging in pretend activities like pretending to be a doctor or assisting with household chores, children learn about different roles and responsibilities and develop empathy, creativity, and problem-solving skills. It's also a great bonding experience between parent and child!

Sheep, camel, bear, giraffe

This game involves placing large pictures of animals in each corner of the room and playing music. When the music stops, children must quickly run to a corner. An adult then calls out the name of an animal, and those in the wrong corner must move to the correct one. The game continues until only one child remains, making it a lively and interactive activity that enhances children's cognitive skills and physical activity.

"Simon says"

This game is suitable for all ages and requires no special equipment or setup. It enhances a child's attention and focus. One person acts as the leader and instructs the others. For example, the leader might say, "Simon says put your hand on your head," and participants must follow. However, if the leader omits "Simon says" and only gives the instruction, those who comply are out of the game. Variations can include using the child's name hosting the party, such as "John says..."

Memory game

This enjoyable game serves as a memory exercise for children. Start by displaying twelve pictures of various items on a board for a brief period before hiding them. Then, give the children a few minutes to recall the pictures from memory. The child who remembers the most pictures wins. You can divide the children into two teams and play competitively for added excitement.

How many names can you come up with?

In this game, you only need a ball or a similar object. Have the children sit in a circle and give the ball to one child who becomes the first player. Then, specify a category of birds or animals (farm animals, zoo animals, pets, etc.), and count to 5. The player must name an animal from that category within that time frame. If they make a mistake, they are out of the game. Pass the ball to another child and continue in this manner. The last player remaining in the game is declared the winner.

Will it fly or not?

Children love birds and animals, but do they know them?

Gather the children in front of you in a semicircle, and then mention the names of various animals and birds. If it's a creature that flies, it should raise its arms and mimic flapping wings. If the creature doesn't fly, they must keep their arms still. Any child who makes a mistake is out of the game; the winner is the last remaining.

Matching

This game is both thrilling and enjoyable for children. Prepare printed pictures of various items, ensuring you have two copies of each picture. Scatter, one set of pictures, face down on the ground while keeping the other set with you. Show the children one picture at a time and have them find its matching pair among the scattered pictures. Repeat this process for each picture, encouraging them to find the matching pairs. Below are some examples of pictures that you can photocopy and use for this game.

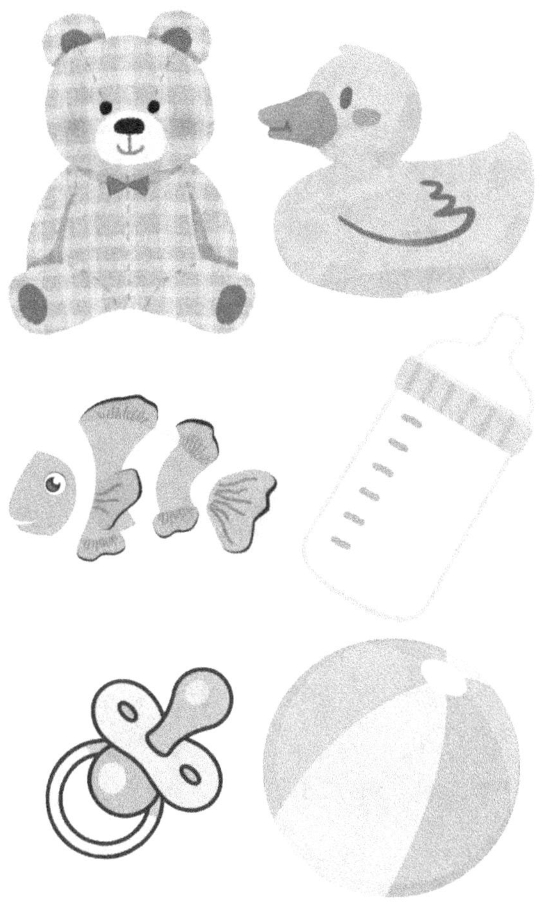

Who or what is this?

In this activity, one child draws or selects a picture and places it face-down on a card. The other children take turns asking you questions that can be answered with "yes" or "no" to determine what is depicted in the drawing. You can use pictures of animals, food, or other items. Here are some examples of pictures that you can use for this activity:

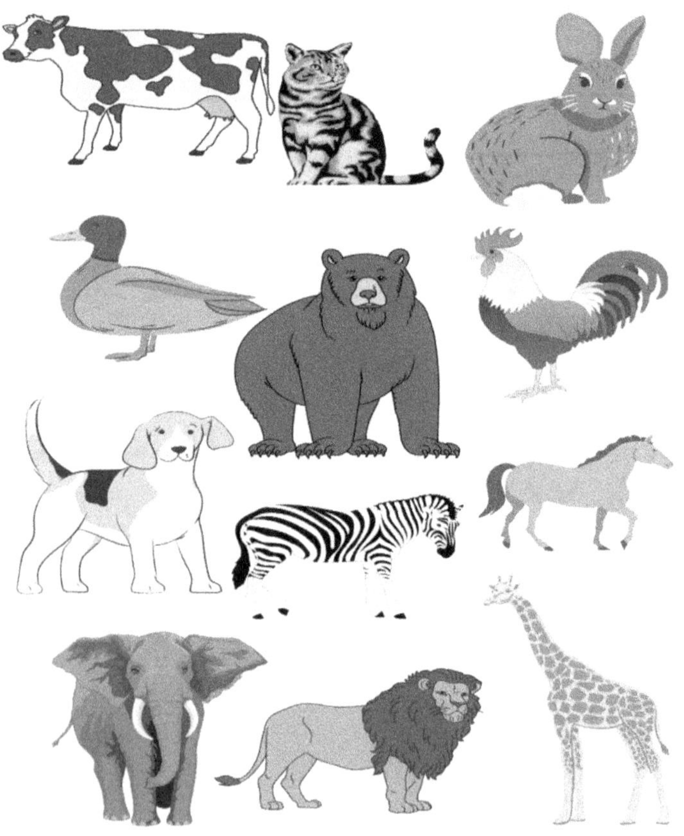

Spontaneous play

Allowing children to run freely or play with a ball outside of structured games with rules provides them with spontaneous playtime to release excess energy and enjoy movement. Give your child the freedom to run in the garden or encourage them to play with a ball. You can join them in a simple, unstructured game of catch by throwing the ball to each other.

Racing

Line up the children and stand some distance away. Tell them that whoever reaches you first will receive a prize or be the winner. This game encourages children to run as fast as possible, promoting their physical development and keeping their bodies healthy and active.

Riding bikes

For children aged 2 to 4 years, bikes should ideally have training wheels to prevent the child from falling off. The child must ride their bike only under adult supervision during this stage. In some countries or regions, cycling helmets are mandatory and highly recommended to prevent head injuries in children.

Pushing and pulling toys

Children derive great enjoyment from toys like tractors or horses with wheels that they can push along, especially when learning to stand and walk. Toys that make noises are preferable, as they add an extra level of interest for the child.

Drawing and coloring

Most children are naturally inclined to draw or scribble with colors, allowing them to express themselves and their emotions. It's important to praise your child each time they finish a drawing, coloring, or even a simple scribble, and encourage them to continue honing their skills. You can assist them in brainstorming drawing ideas and even draw some pictures for them yourself. Teaching them about colors can also be a fun and educational activity. Children often enjoy displaying their artwork prominently in the house, where parents can offer positive feedback and encouragement. Avoid comparing your child's drawings to those of others, as this could potentially discourage them.

Modeling clay or play dough

Engaging in creative play with modeling clay or play dough is beneficial for children's development. Homemade play dough is preferable as it eliminates exposure to chemical substances often found in store-bought modeling clay.

Crafting objects with modeling clay or play dough is a beloved activity among children. To ensure safety, it's important to communicate to the child that the clay or dough is not edible and adult supervision is advisable. After playtime, remind the child to thoroughly wash their hands. To minimize mess, consider using a plastic mat or allowing the child to play with the clay or dough in an uncarpeted area of the house, as pieces dropped and trodden into the carpet can be difficult to remove.

Playdough recipe

To make homemade play dough, you'll need:

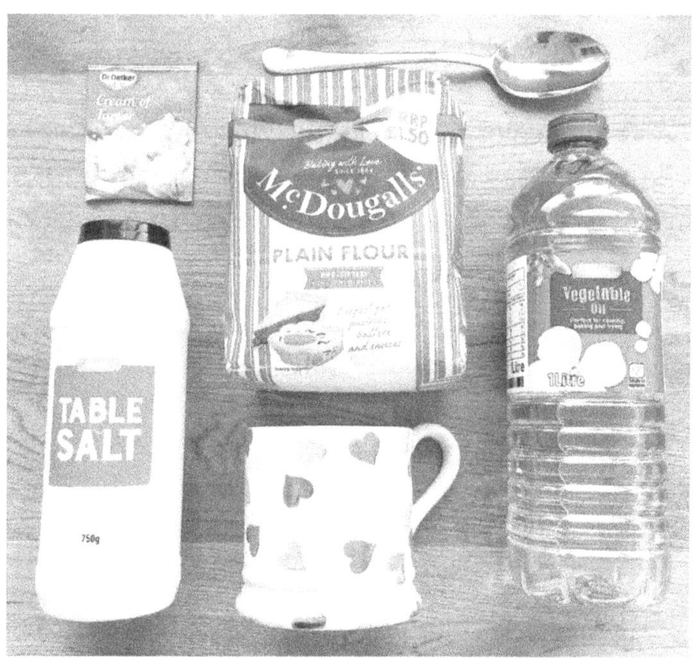

- 1 cup white flour
- 1/2 cup salt
- 2 tablespoons cream of tartar (usually found in the spice section)
- 1 tablespoon oil
- 1 cup water
- Food coloring

Instructions:

- Mix the first 4 ingredients in a pan.
- Add water and mix well.
- Cook over medium heat, stirring constantly, for 3–5 minutes. The dough will become difficult to stir and form a "clump."
- Remove from the stove and knead for 5 minutes. Add food coloring during the kneading process.
- Store the play dough in a covered plastic container or plastic sandwich bag. It will keep for a long time.

No Cook Play Dough Recipe

Ingredients:

- 1 cup of flour
- 1 cup of boiling water
- 2 tablespoons of cream of tartar
- 1/2 cup of salt
- 1 tablespoon of oil

Directions:

- Mix all the ingredients together in a bowl. Be careful, as the mixture can be quite hot due to the boiling water.
- Stir until the ingredients are well combined, forming a dough-like consistency.
- Allow the mixture to cool before handling.
- Once cooled, the play dough is ready for creative play!

Note

Store the play dough in a plastic container with a lid or wrap it tightly to keep it fresh and prevent it from drying out. This will help preserve its texture and usability for future play sessions.

Adding color and scent

Adding food coloring to the play dough mix allows you to create dough of different colors. Some mothers also recommend adding vanilla or cinnamon to the mix to impart a pleasant scent to the play dough, enhancing the sensory experience for children.

Suggested things to make with modeling clay or play dough

Here are some suggested shapes to make with modeling clay or play dough:

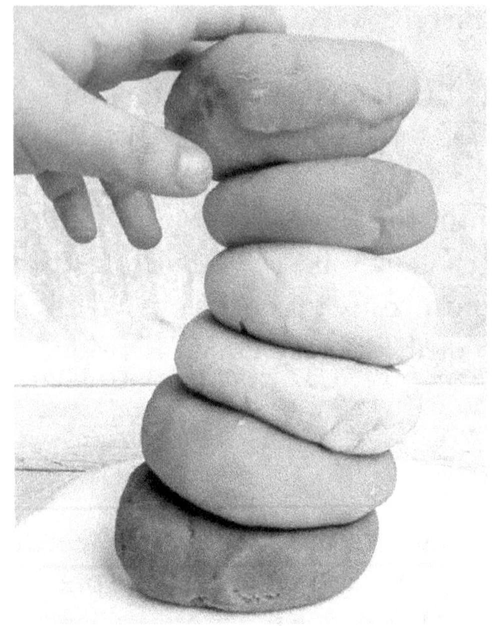

- Basic Shapes: Circle, square, triangle, rectangle
- Animals: Dog, cat, fish, bird
- Objects: Car, boat, house, tree
- Food: Apple, banana, pizza, ice cream cone
- Nature: Sun, cloud, flower, star

Show your child these shapes and help him copy them using modeling clay or play dough. It's a great way to encourage creativity and fine motor skills development.

Nursery rhymes are beloved by children as they provide both entertainment and educational value, especially when they reflect the child's daily experiences, family life, or surroundings like animals and plants. These rhymes also instill positive behaviors in children by incorporating encouraging words about honesty, regular prayer, and other virtues.

Children particularly enjoy rhymes featuring familiar animals or birds. It's important to ensure that the language used in the rhymes is simple and the sentences are short for easy comprehension. Rhymes should be cheerful and amusing, allowing children to follow the rhythm. Traditional rhymes and songs from one's own culture can be used, and some may even adapt traditional rhymes to better suit contemporary values.

Examples of some nursery rhymes or songs that mothers can teach to their children

Disclaimer: all lyrics are properties of their respective owners and are provided for informational and educational purposes only. For more nursery rhymes and songs, visit **bussongs.com**

"Twinkle, Twinkle, Little Star"

This song talks about a little star shining brightly in the sky. It encourages children to wonder about the stars and the universe.

"Twinkle, twinkle, little star, how I wonder what you are! Up above the world so high, like a diamond in the sky. Twinkle, twinkle, little star, how I wonder what you are! "

(https://www.bussongs.com)

"Old MacDonald Had a Farm"

This song introduces various farm animals and the sounds they make. It's a fun way for children to learn about farm life.

"Old MacDonald had a farm, E-I-E-I-O. And on his farm, he had a cow, E-I-E-I-O. With a moo-moo here and a moo-moo there, here a moo, there a moo, everywhere a moo-moo."

(https://www.bussongs.com)

"The Wheels on the Bus"

This song describes the various parts of a bus and what they do, accompanied by fun actions. It's interactive and encourages participation.

"The wheels on the bus go round and round, round and round, round and round. The wheels on the bus go round and round, all through the town."

(https://www.bussongs.com)

"If You're Happy and You Know It"

This song encourages children to express their happiness through actions like clapping their hands, stomping their feet, and shouting "Hooray!" It's a joyful and energetic song.

"If you're happy and you know it, clap your hands (clap, clap). If you're happy and you know it, clap your hands (clap, clap). If you're happy and you know it, then your face will surely show it. If you're happy and you know it, , clap your hands (clap, clap)!'"

(https://www.bussongs.com)

"The Itsy-bitsy Spider"

This song describes the journey of a spider as it climbs up a water spout, gets washed away by rain, and then climbs up again. It's a fun and repetitive rhyme.

"The itsy-bitsy spider climbed up the water spout. Down came the rain and washed the spider out. Out came the sun and dried up all the rain, and the itsy-bitsy spider climbed up the spout again."

"Humpty Dumpty"

This nursery rhyme tells the story of Humpty Dumpty, a character who falls off a wall and breaks into pieces. It's a classic rhyme with a simple storyline.

"Humpty Dumpty sat on a wall. Humpty Dumpty had a great fall. All the king's horses and all the king's men couldn't put Humpty together again."

(https://www.bussongs.com)

Children enjoy hearing stories, often referred to as "fairy tales," from their mothers. Using picture books can make the child's stories more vivid and engaging. These stories can teach customs, behaviors, or religious practices like prayer and obedience to parents.

However, it's important to avoid scary stories, such as tales about ghosts or dangerous animals, that might frighten the child. Here's an example of a story about the importance of dental hygiene:

Once, Peter bought some sweets on his way home from school and ate them without brushing his teeth. That night, he dreamed of seeing an evil worm attacking weak teeth, attracted by candy. Fortunately, the smart teeth quickly grabbed a toothbrush and toothpaste, washed away the candy, and defeated the worm. Peter woke up and immediately brushed his teeth, realizing the importance of dental hygiene. From that day on, he cared for his teeth, never forgetting to brush them properly.

Froebel describes the kindergarten as a nurturing environment where young children can grow and develop, much like flowers in a garden tended by a caring gardener. The kindergarten teacher's role is to facilitate this growth by nurturing the children's inner feelings and allowing them to express themselves through various activities and play.

The purpose of nursery schools and kindergartens is to prepare children to transition to elementary school, ensuring a smooth adjustment from home to formal education. These institutions allow children to freely explore their interests, abilities, and potential. They aim to foster new skills and experiences while encouraging the child's collaboration, cooperation, self-reliance, and self-confidence.

Modern educational practices prioritize the child's autonomy and engagement in self-directed activities, emphasizing free play over coercion or force. The focus is on flexibility, innovation, revitalization, and inclusiveness. Effective implementation of these principles requires qualified teachers who are passionate about their work and capable of nurturing children with love, kindness, and patience.

Maria Montessori highlights children's innate curiosity and exploratory tendencies right from birth. She argues that kindergartens should cater to this intrinsic desire for discovery by providing an environment that aligns with the child's developmental needs. Montessori recognizes that children progress through distinct stages of growth, each characterized by its own set of requirements and milestones.

Throughout the initial three years of life, children predominantly learn through their physical senses and absorb information from their surroundings. Linguistic development takes precedence between the ages of one and a half to three years. From two to four years old, children commence refining their motor skills and grasping concepts of order and sequence.

Sensory perception undergoes improvement from two and a half to six years old. Writing preparation typically commences around three and a half to four and a half years old, while tactile sensitivity refines from four to four and a half years old. Reading readiness emerges between four and a half to five years old.

Montessori advocates for establishing a stimulating educational environment in kindergartens, complete with diverse educational tools to support children's intellectual, psychological, and physical development.

Kindergarten is a pivotal educational phase with its unique philosophy and objectives, focusing on nurturing individuality, fostering independent thought, and promoting adaptability. Additionally, kindergarten endeavors to instill healthy habits, impart social skills, cultivate an appreciation for music, beauty, and nature, and foster a sense of altruism and collaboration among children.

Selecting Suitable Daycare or Nursery School

Teachers' qualifications

One of the critical aspects of nursery schools and daycares is the educational competence of the teachers responsible for the children's learning and care. These educators serve as surrogate mothers to the children, guiding them through their first experiences away from home. The child's educational development hinges largely on the teacher's abilities and qualifications.

Regrettably, some nursery schools and kindergartens overlook the importance of hiring highly qualified teachers. However, the teacher's influence extends beyond mere instruction; they serve as role models whom children often emulate in character, behavior, and demeanor.

Therefore, considering the teacher's character, values, emotions, and habits is just as crucial as evaluating their professional background, experience, and technical skills.

Location

The ideal nursery location is close to the child's home, facilitating easy access by foot. Furthermore, it's advantageous for the nursery to be situated away from bustling markets, noisy environments, industrial areas, and main roads to ensure the child's safety and minimize exposure to pollutants and traffic hazards. Ideally, the nursery should be located among residential areas to provide the child a comforting and familiar environment. Additionally, surrounded by gardens or green spaces allows the child to appreciate and interact with natural beauty, enhancing their overall experience.

Size

The nursery's size should be tailored to accommodate the number and ages of the children it serves and the variety of indoor and outdoor activities they will participate in. Additionally, the building should include essential facilities such as administrative offices, meeting rooms, kitchens, washrooms, and medical examination rooms. Sufficient space is necessary to allow children the freedom to play and move around comfortably without feeling cramped.

Building

The design of the building should prioritize health considerations, including sun exposure and wind direction. Positioning the building to face north in hot climates can help mitigate sun exposure. Adequate access to natural light and airflow is essential for the well-being of the children and should be carefully incorporated into the building's design.

Playrooms and gardens

The nursery should feature a grassy area as well as a clean sand area, along with ample play equipment such as swings and slides. These outdoor spaces provide opportunities for children to engage in active play and exploration, contributing to their physical development and well-being.

Health and psychological services

The nursery should incorporate health services, including a designated first aid room, access to natural remedies, and an office for a social worker. These provisions ensure the well-being and safety of the children attending the nursery, offering physical and emotional support as needed.

Health and safety concerns

The mother needs to consider the safety and appropriateness of eating utensils. It's crucial to avoid glass utensils that may break or plastic ones that can interact with food. Stainless steel utensils are the best choice for safety. Additionally, she should ensure that play equipment is safe and that art supplies like crayons and paint are non-toxic to prevent any harm to the child.

Is it the role of the nursery school or kindergarten to teach the child how to read and write?

Although the child is mentally ready to absorb new words and expand their vocabulary, their muscle control is not fully developed, especially the fine motor skills required for proper pen grip and control. Additionally, their nervous system and vision are not yet mature enough for reading and focusing. Attempting to teach a child to read and write at this stage is comparable to expecting a five-month-old to stand and walk.

It's important to clarify that the primary aim of nursery school or kindergarten is not to introduce formal reading, writing, or subjects like language, religion, and mathematics. These aspects will be addressed in later academic stages.

Instead, the focus should be on nurturing the child's verbal communication skills, fostering attentiveness, listening ability, and curiosity, instilling a love for books and learning, developing motor skills, and cultivating awareness of the senses.

At this stage, the child can sense, understand, see, and comprehend their surroundings, which lays the foundation for social and emotional harmony and teaches them to respect the wishes and feelings of others. Additionally, it's crucial to impart religious, moral, aesthetic, and patriotic values to help the child distinguish between right and wrong, beauty and ugliness, in their interactions with others.

All of these objectives should be approached as a cohesive and interconnected unit. There can be no prioritization of one goal over another if we aim to foster the child's happiness and readiness to contribute positively to society.

Preparing the child for reading

The goal of preparing the child to read and write does not imply teaching them these skills during the nursery school or kindergarten stage. As previously emphasized, it is not within the scope of nursery school or kindergarten to instruct children in reading and writing. Rather, the primary objective is to enhance the child's cognitive, physical, psychological, social, and linguistic abilities to prepare them for formal schooling, where reading and writing will be introduced.

Therefore, during the kindergarten stage, it is crucial to expand the child's vocabulary in anticipation of reading and to develop the fine motor skills of their hands in preparation for writing.

Parties and trips

These social activities are beloved by children as they bring happiness and a sense of participation in daily life, fostering a feeling of belonging within a larger group. Parties and trips expand a child's vocabulary and provide new experiences that engage their senses and understanding. Such activities promote self-reliance and bolster social bonds with peers.

Dramatic play

Engaging in make-believe and role-playing allows children to express themselves, enhance their discernment, and foster reasoning skills.

Telling stories

Telling stories to children is beneficial as it enhances their vocabulary, fosters imagination, encourages creativity and innovation and cultivates attentive listening skills.

Alphabet games

The use of flashcards is instrumental in teaching the child letters. Write the same letter on several cards, except for one, which displays a different letter. Have the child identify the card with the different letters. This method enhances the child's ability to focus and observe details up close, facilitating later engagement with books and aiding in the development of hand-eye coordination.

Puppets

Puppet shows serve as a method for children to familiarize themselves with various traditions, ideas, and behaviors, aiding their linguistic development.

Preparing children to write

To prepare children for writing, efforts focus on enhancing coordination, improving visual skills, bolstering hand and finger muscle strength, and acquiring correct pen-holding techniques.

Examples of activities that develop the child's skills and help him get ready to write

- Provide the child with pens and paper to encourage initial scribbling, allowing time for familiarization with the tools.
- Progressively instruct the child on proper pen-holding techniques.
- Offer lines for the child to trace with the pen, aiding in skill development, hand-eye coordination, and hand-muscle strengthening.

Examples:
Let your child join the dots to make a straight line

Let your child trace over these lines and shapes with a
pencil or crayon

Disclaimer: The content in this chapter serves informational purposes only and does not replace any medical advice or treatment for any specific medical condition. It is not intended to diagnose, treat, cure, or prevent any particular disease or condition.

The information provided does not substitute the advice of your physician, general practitioner, medical practitioner, or healthcare provider, nor is it meant to diagnose, treat, cure, or prevent any specific disease or condition. Any health concerns or issues should be addressed by consulting your doctor or pediatrician.

Common cold

The common cold is the most frequent illness among young children. Due to their underdeveloped immune systems, children may experience multiple colds in a year until around five. Symptoms typically include a runny nose, watery eyes, sore throat, cough, sneezing, and occasionally a low-grade fever. Over two hundred viruses can impact the upper respiratory tract, leading to cold symptoms. This mild respiratory illness is caused by one of these viruses.

Precautions to avoid spreading viruses

- Encourage consistent handwashing among children, as the cold virus can persist on hands for an extended period, and handshaking is a common means of transmission.
- Instruct the child to promptly dispose of used tissues.
- Ensure thorough cleaning of kitchen utensils, particularly plates, spoons, and cups, especially if a family member is experiencing a cold. This practice helps prevent the virus from spreading to other family members.

Taking care of a child with a cold

- Avoid using antibiotics since there isn't an effective drug to expedite recovery from a cold, and antibiotics don't treat the virus causing the illness.
- Encourage the child to stay hydrated by drinking plenty of fluids.
- Teach the child to blow their nose whenever they feel it's blocked.
- Use a nasal saline spray to alleviate congestion, as it's considered safe and doesn't trigger nasal allergies like some medications might in small children.
- Refrain from giving aspirin to children under twelve if they have the flu, as it can lead to Reye's

syndrome, a potentially fatal condition, and other serious health issues affecting the blood, liver, and brain.

- Maintain a high humidity level in the home, as dry air worsens cold symptoms, contrary to common practices.
- Consult a doctor before administering cough suppressant medicine to the child, as coughing helps clear the airways and prevent further infection.

When should you call the doctor?

- Seek medical attention if the cold persists for over 3 to 4 days.
- Consult a doctor for ear pain or signs of infection.
- If the child's temperature suddenly rises, seek medical advice.
- Seek immediate medical attention if the child's breathing remains abnormal.
- Contact a healthcare provider if there's a loss of appetite or vomiting.
- Consult a doctor in case of stomach pain.
- Seek medical advice if the child experiences severe headaches and continuous crying.

Lastly, I advise the mother to remain patient and take good care of her child, as the cold virus typically persists until the body produces antibodies to eliminate it.

Influenza (flu)

Influenza (flu) is a respiratory illness with symptoms similar to the common cold but is more severe and caused by a different virus. Symptoms include headache, chills, and cough, followed rapidly by fever, loss of appetite, muscle aches, fatigue, runny nose, sneezing, watery eyes, and throat irritation.

Nausea, vomiting, and diarrhea may also occur, especially in children. The most common type is seasonal flu, with cases typically occurring between October and May. Occasionally, there are concerns about different types of flu, such as bird flu and swine flu, caused by new strains of the virus incorporating genes from bird or pig flu strains.

Signs and Symptoms	Influenza	Cold
Fever	Usually present	Rare
Aches	Usual, often severe	Slight
Chills	Fairly common	Uncommon
Tiredness	Moderate to severe	Mild
Symptom onset	Symptoms can appear within 3 to 6 hours	Symptoms appear gradually
Coughing	Dry, unproductive cough	Hacking, productive cough
Sneezing	Uncommon	Common
Stuffy nose	Uncommon	Common
Sore throat	Uncommon	Common
Chest discomfort	Often severe	Mild to moderate
Headache	Common	Uncommon

Is it a cold or flu?

The chart above shows the main differences between
the two:

Treating flu

Because the flu is caused by a virus, antibiotics won't
aid in treatment or speed up recovery. Frequent rest
and fluids are typically recommended for the sick child,
and acetaminophen (paracetamol) may help alleviate
fever and muscle aches. Aspirin should be avoided in
children as it can lead to Reyes syndrome, a potentially
fatal condition.

In many countries, people are encouraged to get an
annual vaccination, known as the "flu shot," for
protection against influenza. Additionally, there are
further precautions to guard against the flu and other
infectious illnesses:

The World Health Organization recommends taking
certain precautionary measures to safeguard yourself
and your child from the flu and other illnesses. These
precautions include:

Influenza
How you can protect yourself and others

Remember to:

- Use a tissue when coughing or sneezing.
- Dispose of the tissue immediately in the trash after use.
- Always wash your hands with soap and water.
- If you experience any flu symptoms, promptly visit the doctor.
- Maintain a distance of at least 1 meter from others if you have flu symptoms.
- Refrain from leaving your home and going to work, school, or crowded places if you have flu symptoms.
- Avoid hugging, kissing, or shaking hands when greeting others.
- Do not touch your eyes, nose, or mouth without washing your hands.

Most children suffer from occasional bouts of diarrhea.

Diarrhea is characterized by the transformation of solid stools into liquid or watery stools, with the child defecating more than three times in one day. It's particularly prevalent in children aged six months to two years but can also occur in infants under six months old, especially if they are bottle-fed rather than breastfed.

Causes of diarrhea

- Ingesting pathogens through the mouth, such as viruses, bacteria, and parasites, can lead to diarrhea. This can occur via contaminated milk, water, food, or contaminated items like bottles and teats. Poor sanitation and exposure to garbage can also introduce these viruses into the environment.
- Diarrhea may result as a side effect of certain medications, such as antibiotics like penicillin, or from administering excessive doses of vitamins to the child.
- Diarrhea can also be a symptom of various illnesses, including infections caused by viruses, bacteria, and parasites.

Symptoms that may accompany diarrhea

- Vomiting is considered one of the primary symptoms.
- Severe redness around the anus.
- High temperature.
- Abdominal pain.

Dehydration

Dehydration is recognized as one of the most serious complications of diarrhea. Therefore, it's crucial to closely monitor the child whenever they have diarrhea and ensure prompt treatment for this symptom.

Symptoms of dehydration

- Increased thirst - the more thirsty the child feels, the more likely it indicates dehydration.
- Dryness in the mouth and on the lips.
- Sunken eyes.
- Loss of flexibility in the skin; you can assess skin flexibility by lightly pinching the skin on the stomach or neck between two fingers; if it is slow to return to normal, this is a sign of dehydration.
- Loss of appetite.
- High temperature.
- Abnormal drowsiness or apathy.
- Not urinating for six consecutive hours.
- Loss of balance.
- Rapid heartbeat.
- Lack of tears.

Treating dehydration

To prepare a 1-liter solution using salt, sugar, and water at home, follow this recipe:

Ingredients:

- Six level teaspoons of sugar
- Half-level teaspoon of salt
- One liter of clean drinking or boiled water (cooled) - approximately 5 cupfuls (each cup about 200 ml)

Preparation Method:

- Stir the mixture until the salt and sugar dissolve.

This homemade oral rehydration solution is an efficient and effective remedy for watery diarrhea. Here's how to make it:

Ingredients:

- 1/2 to 1 cup precooked baby rice cereal or 1½ tablespoons of granulated sugar
- 2 cups of water
- 1/2 teaspoon salt

Instructions:

- Mix the rice cereal (or sugar), water, and salt together until the mixture thickens but is still drinkable.
- Offer the mixture often by spoon and provide as much as the child will accept, aiming to replace the lost fluids. If one cup is lost, give a cup.
- Even if the child is vomiting, offer small amounts (2-3 teaspoons) every few minutes.
- Bananas or other non-sweetened mashed fruits can provide potassium.
- Continue feeding children when sick and breastfeeding if the child is being breastfed.

10 Things you should know about rehydrating a child.

Here's a guide to preparing and administering an oral rehydration solution (ORS) at home:

- Wash your hands with soap and water before preparing the solution.
- In a clean pot, mix six level teaspoons of sugar and half a teaspoon of salt or one packet of Oral Rehydration Salts (ORS) (20.5 grams) with one liter of clean drinking or boiled water (cooled). Stir the mixture until all the contents dissolve.
- Wash your and baby's hands with soap and water before feeding the solution.
- Offer the sick child as much of the solution as needed, in small amounts frequently.
- Give the child alternative fluids like breast milk and juices.
- Continue to offer solids if the child is four months or older.
- If the child still requires ORS after 24 hours, prepare a fresh solution.
- Remember, ORS does not stop diarrhea; it prevents the body from dehydrating. Diarrhea will typically stop on its own.
- If the child vomits, wait ten minutes, and then offer ORS again. Vomiting usually subsides.

- If diarrhea increases and/or vomiting persists, take the child to a health clinic for further evaluation and treatment.

Healthy nutrition for your child

Infants

Mother's milk contains numerous beneficial substances that aid in restoring the lining of the intestines and provide resistance against bacteria. Therefore, the best thing you can give your baby when they have diarrhea is the mother's milk in whatever amount is possible, supplemented with an electrolyte solution to replenish lost fluids.

For bottle-fed babies, some doctors consider it preferable to switch from formula milk to electrolyte solution for between twelve and twenty-four hours to replace lost fluids from the body. After this period, you can resume giving the baby formula milk.

Older children

On the first day, if the child experiences dehydration, it's preferable to offer the following foods: banana, apple, rice, and toast. Then, gradually introduce other foods based on the child's appetite on the second and third days. It's important to avoid foods high in sugar and fats, such as ice cream, fried foods, and dairy products, for three to seven days.

Prevention of diarrhea

- Thoroughly wash hands before preparing food and clean fruits, vegetables, herbs, and grains before cooking. To be eaten raw, they must be washed even more carefully.
- Wash vessels and utensils for cooking and eating thoroughly before using them.
- Maintain cleanliness in the house to prevent insects, as transmission of viruses by flies and cockroaches can cause diarrhea.
- Reheat cooked food properly before eating to kill any germs that may have formed during storage. Reheating food properly means it should reach a temperature of at least 70°C.
- Feed your child healthy foods; consider breastfeeding when they are young and provide a balanced diet as they age.
- Ensure your child is vaccinated against contagious diseases to prevent illness.

The danger of kissing your small child on his mouth

Kissing the child in his mouth can be very dangerous, especially in the first three months when his immune system is not fully developed. The kiss from either parent, if they are suffering from any disease, can transmit various illnesses to the child.

This can lead to fungal infections on the tongue or the spread of bacteria like staphylococcus, resulting in throat and mouth infections, including tonsillitis.

Serious complications such as heart issues or repeated kidney infections may arise as the child grows, particularly by the age of two. One disease that can be spread via kissing is cerebrospinal fever, caused by bacteria naturally occurring in the human mouth. Doctors recommend kissing the child's hand or forehead to minimize risks, as bacteria die quickly on these surfaces.

Food allergies

How can I know if my child is allergic to a certain type of food?

Detecting food allergies in infants and young children involves observing reactions such as skin rashes, hives, eczema, red spots, or swelling in the lips or eyelids following the consumption of specific foods.

Anaphylactic shock

Anaphylactic shock, also referred to as anaphylaxis, is a swift and severe allergic reaction that can be deeply alarming for parents when experienced by young children. It begins when the immune system mistakenly reacts to a harmless substance, releasing histamine and other chemicals that trigger a range of symptoms, some of which may pose life-threatening risks.

Symptoms in toddlers encompass swelling of the skin, lips, throat, tongue, or face, wheezing or severe breathing difficulties, rapid or irregular heartbeat, hives, dizziness, fainting, loss of consciousness, nausea, vomiting, abdominal cramps, diarrhea, extremely pale or blue skin, sweating, redness, confusion, and more.

These symptoms typically arise within two hours following exposure to the allergen, though they can manifest within minutes or up to four hours later.

What should I do if my toddler seems to be Having a severe allergic reaction?

Immediately call for an ambulance if your toddler experiences difficulty breathing or loses consciousness. Lay him down with his feet elevated to minimize the risk of shock, and try to keep him calm by speaking reassuringly and maintaining your own composure. Do not administer antihistamines if your child has trouble breathing or swallowing, as it may cause choking.

Upon arrival, paramedics will likely administer an epinephrine injection to halt the allergic reaction swiftly. Epinephrine boosts heart function, relaxes airway muscles, reduces swelling, and enhances blood flow to vital areas like the heart and brain. Your toddler will then be transported to the hospital for examination and monitoring for any delayed reactions. Hospital doctors can help identify the trigger and may recommend follow-up with a pediatric allergist.

Anaphylaxis is a potentially life-threatening condition, and even a mild initial episode does not guarantee subsequent milder reactions. Avoiding trigger foods is crucial, and your doctor may advise carrying an EpiPen for emergency use.

It's important to inform caregivers and teachers, and in many cases, keeping an EpiPen at home and at daycare or school is recommended.

What can I do for my child who has a food allergy?

To identify which foods are triggering your child's allergic symptoms and confirm whether they have an allergy, it's essential to observe and experiment from the earliest stages. According to the American Medical Encyclopedia, allergies manifest as a heightened immune system response to typically harmless substances.

Keep track of foods that elicit allergic reactions and share this list with a specialist. The doctor may conduct skin or blood tests to pinpoint the specific allergen causing the reaction.

This proactive approach allows for early detection and effective management of food allergies in children.

Foods that children are most commonly allergic to

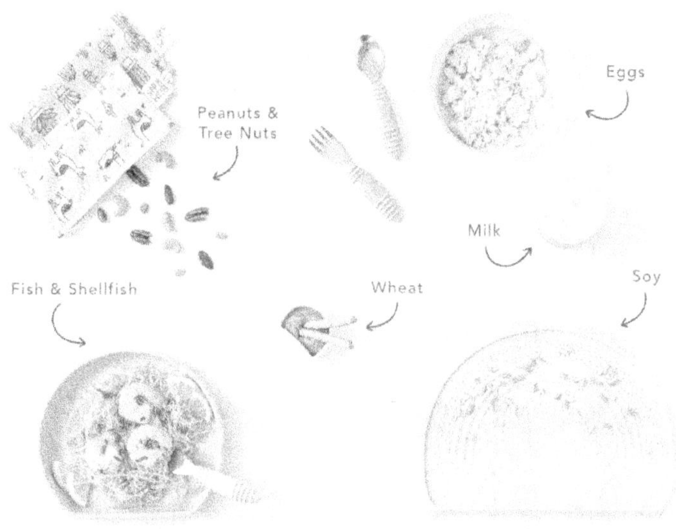

Chocolate, cow's milk, eggs, fish, shellfish, peanuts, and tree nuts are among the foods that commonly trigger allergic reactions in children. However, this doesn't mean your child must avoid these foods altogether. Instead, monitoring your child closely each time they consume these items is crucial to observe any allergic reactions. Children may often outgrow allergies to certain foods, such as eggs. However, in severe, potentially life-threatening cases like peanut allergy, complete avoidance of the food is necessary. Parents must remain vigilant as the allergen may be concealed in foods like cookies and processed dishes.

What should I do if my child has an allergy to milk?

In this scenario, you can opt for types of milk from which the cow's milk protein has been eliminated. Additionally, alternative "milk" is derived from soy, rice, almonds, and other sources, which could serve as suitable substitutes if the child isn't allergic to the ingredients they are made from.

Treating food allergies

The most effective approach to treating food allergies involves:

- Identifying the substance triggering the allergy.
- Removing this substance from the child's diet, with potential alternatives discussed with the doctor.
- Breastfeeding during the first year may offer protection against food allergies.
- Introducing complementary foods gradually alongside breast milk while delaying the introduction of common allergy-inducing foods like eggs, fish, and chocolate until the child is 9 to 12 months old.

- Recognizing that in many cases, food allergies in children become less severe and may disappear as the child grows older.

Asthma

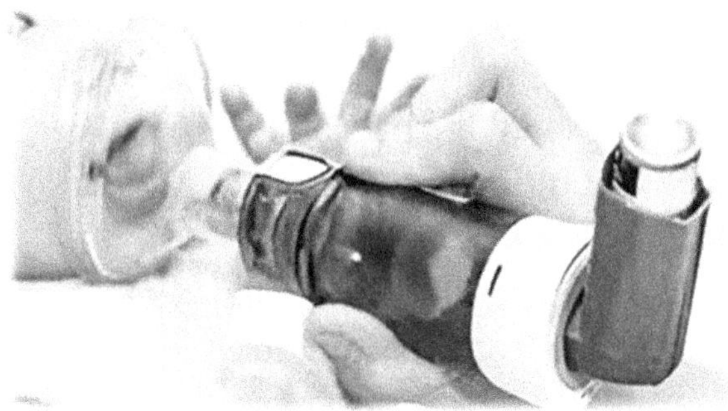

Asthma is a common chronic inflammatory disease affecting the airways, which can be triggered by various factors such as viruses, dust, pollen, medications, dampness, climate changes, or allergens. It's often hereditary and typically diagnosed in children after the age of one, with a higher prevalence in boys compared to girls. Most children with asthma experience improvement as they enter adolescence.

symptoms

Symptoms of asthma include difficulty breathing, wheezing, tightness in the chest, trouble sleeping, and nighttime coughing.

Prevention and treatment strategies include:

- Medications prescribed by the doctor to widen the airways.
- In cases where airway-widening medications aren't effective, short-term steroid use may be recommended until the child can inhale or take medication orally.
- Calming the child during asthma episodes.
- Regular vacuuming reduces dust and other irritants in the child's environment.
- Avoiding contact with individuals who have colds and refraining from kissing the child on the mouth.
- Maintaining a smoke-free environment indoors.
- Washing bed sheets and blankets in hot water at least once a month, with pillowcases washed weekly.
- Avoid exposure to car exhaust and smoke.
- Monitoring and identifying triggers for asthma attacks, especially severe ones, by observing when they occur.

Chickenpox

Chickenpox is caused by the Varicella zoster virus and is highly contagious, primarily transmitted from one child to another. It typically affects children, with an incubation period ranging from two to three weeks, averaging around fourteen days.

The patient remains contagious from the day before symptoms onset until six days after symptoms appear.

Symptoms of chickenpox

- There is a slight increase in temperature (38°C).
- The eyes become red, and there is an increase in secretions.
- Some children experience tiredness, exhaustion, headache, and a mild cough.
- About twenty-four hours later, a skin rash develops, consisting of small red bumps resembling pimples or insect bites. These bumps become blisters filled with clear liquid, primarily appearing on the face and torso. Once the blisters break, they leave behind open sores that eventually crust over and form dry scabs.

Is this illness contagious?

Chickenpox is highly contagious. A child with chickenpox can spread the disease from approximately 2 days before the rash appears until all the blisters have crusted over.

Ways in which the disease is spread

- Transmission occurs through airborne particles released during talking, sneezing, or coughing.
- Direct contact with the skin or touching a blister or its fluid can also spread the disease.

- Mixing healthy children with those who have the illness can lead to transmission.

Ways in which the disease is spread

Typically, chickenpox is not severe in most children; however, it can pose a risk for those with weakened immune systems or who are taking immune-suppressing medication. In pregnant women, chickenpox can be severe, and if contracted early in pregnancy, there is a slight risk of harm to the fetus.

Prevention and treatment of chickenpox

- There is a vaccine available to provide protection against chickenpox.
- It's important to isolate the sick child as much as possible for about a week after the rash first appears.
- Cams like calamine lotion can help alleviate itching and prevent contamination of the spots. However, it's essential not to overapply, as this can dry out the skin and worsen itching.
- Trim the child's nails to minimize the risk of complications from scratching.
- Avoid giving aspirin to a child with chickenpox. Instead, acetaminophen (Paracetamol) may provide some relief.
- Antibiotics cannot treat chickenpox because it is caused by a virus.

- Children at risk, including those receiving immune-suppressing drugs, may receive varicella zoster immune globulin after exposure to chickenpox to reduce its severity.

Poliomyelitis

Poliomyelitis, known as polio, is a viral infection caused by the poliovirus. It typically spreads more frequently during late summer and early fall. This virus impacts the central nervous system; its severity can vary from severe to mild. In some cases, it can lead to permanent paralysis in certain body parts.

Ways in which polio is transmitted

- It spreads from the infected person through airborne particles released during coughing, sneezing, or speaking.
- Additionally, it can be transmitted through contamination of food or drinks with particles from the stools of an infected person, facilitated by flies and other insects.

Incubation period

The incubation period of polio ranges from 3 to 21 days and can sometimes extend beyond that duration.

Symptoms of polio

Symptoms encompass high fever, headache, stiffness in the back and neck, asymmetrical weakness in various muscles, sensitivity to touch, difficulty swallowing, muscle pain, loss of superficial and deep reflexes, paresthesia (pins and needles), irritability, constipation or difficulty urinating. In severe cases, paralysis of the muscles of the respiratory system may occur, potentially leading to death if artificial means of respiration, like an "iron lung," are not utilized.

Prevention and treatment

- Compulsory vaccination and booster shots are required at two, four, and six months.
- Isolation of the patient is essential to prevent the spread of the disease to others.
- Physiotherapy provided in the hospital aims to aid in rehabilitating muscle fibers affected by the disease.

Whooping cough (pertussis)

Whooping cough, caused by the Bordetella pertussis bacterium, is a contagious bacterial infection. It spreads through direct contact with the patient's mouth, airborne particles from sneezing or coughing, or touching objects belonging to the patient. The main symptom is a persistent and severe cough, often ending with a distinctive "whooping" sound during inhalation.

Incubation period

The incubation period of whooping cough ranges from four to twenty-one days, with an average duration of seven days.

Symptoms of whooping cough

- Persistent episodes of coughing that occur frequently and are marked by the distinctive "whoop" sound, which gives the illness its common name.
- Elevated body temperature.
- Breathing in with a noise resembling that of a rooster.
- Cyanosis is indicated by bluish skin discoloration during coughing due to decreased oxygen levels in the blood.

Most serious complications of whooping cough

- Onset of pneumonia, 3 to 5 weeks after the initial illness.
- Development of umbilical hernia or rectal prolapse.
- Inflammation of the meninges and brain, presenting as convulsions and loss of consciousness.
- Bronchitis.

Prevention and treatment of whooping cough

- Administer the DTaP vaccine at two, four, and six months, followed by booster shots.
- Isolating the patient to prevent illness transmission to other children.
- Using erythromycin, an antibiotic, to shorten the period of infectiousness and minimize the spread of the disease.
- Ensuring proper ventilation in the patient's room and providing good nutrition.

Measles

Measles, a viral infection of the respiratory system, is highly contagious and poses a significant risk to children, as one in fifteen affected children will experience complications.

The virus is transmitted through airborne particles from the nose and mouth of an infected individual.

Incubation period

The incubation period for measles ranges from ten to fourteen days, during which the virus can be transmitted both before and after the appearance of the characteristic rash.

Symptoms of measles

- Elevated body temperature.
- Symptoms include sneezing, coughing, blocked nose, and swollen eyes.
- The rash emerges approximately 4 to 5 days later, starting on the forehead and cheeks before spreading to the face, extremities, stomach, and back.
- The temperature escalates notably alongside increased coughing, eye swelling, and light sensitivity.

Prevention and treatment

- Adhering to the recommended schedule for MMR vaccination as per local medical guidelines.
- Keeping the patient isolated from healthy individuals as much as possible.
- Ensuring complete bed rest in a dimly lit room.
- Providing the child with ample fluids and a well-balanced diet.

- Administering acetaminophen (Paracetamol) or ibuprofen to alleviate fever symptoms; avoiding aspirin for children.
- Reserving antibiotics for cases of secondary bacterial infection only.
- Avoid exposure to sunlight or excessive heat.
- Taking measures to prevent infection of the eye membranes.

Rubella (German measles)

Rubella, commonly known as "German measles," is a distinct viral illness from measles despite their similar names. Primarily affecting the skin and lymph nodes, rubella typically results in a mild rash in young children. However, the primary concern arises when rubella affects pregnant women, as it can lead to severe defects in the developing fetus. The rubella virus is transmitted through airborne particles from an infected individual.

Incubation period

The incubation period for rubella ranges from fourteen to twenty days from the initial exposure to the illness.

Symptoms of German measles

- Symptoms resembling the common cold include coughing, sneezing, blocked nose, and high temperature.

- Rash persists for three days.
- Possible presence of red spots in the mouth.
- Skin may exhibit very small flakes where the rash occurred.

Prevention and treatment

- Immunization using the MMR vaccine.
- Isolation of the patient.
- There isn't a targeted treatment for rubella; efforts are directed towards mitigating symptom severity if necessary.

Rheumatic fever

This inflammatory condition arises from an infection with Streptococcus bacteria, typically originating from the patients if they experience recurring throat and tonsil infections. It commonly manifests in children aged between six and twelve years.

Causes of rheumatic fever

- Rheumatic fever can arise due to an abnormal immune response in individuals with a genetic predisposition, where the immune system targets various body parts beyond just the Streptococcus bacteria.
- Rheumatic fever might occur following a respiratory infection with no symptoms.

Is rheumatic fever a hereditary disease?

No, it's not hereditary, but genetic factors may increase susceptibility to this disease.

Is rheumatic fever contagious?

Rheumatic fever is considered non-contagious. However, what can be contagious is the Streptococcus throat infection. Overcrowding in schools, homes, and marketplaces contributes to the spread of infection with this bacterium.

Symptoms of rheumatic fever

- Elevated body temperature.
- Polyarthritis is characterized by temporary migrating inflammation of the large joints, typically initiating in the legs and progressing upwards.
- Carditis, involving heart muscle inflammation, represents the most severe symptom.
- Decreased appetite and fatigue with minimal exertion.
- Rash may manifest on the trunk or arms.

Blood tests for diagnosis of rheumatic fever

Blood tests serve as a diagnostic tool for rheumatic fever, complementing the symptoms outlined earlier. While obtaining a throat swab to detect Streptococcus bacteria through lab cultivation isn't considered diagnostically useful due to the bacteria's reduction in the throat during illness onset, it's crucial to note that the presence of Streptococcus bacteria in the blood doesn't automatically indicate a diagnosis of rheumatic fever. Instead, it signifies the immune system's production of antibodies in response to the infection.

Prevention and treatment

- Avoiding crowded areas and enhancing the child's living environment.
- Providing appropriate treatment if the child experiences recurrent throat and tonsil infections.
- Seeking guidance from the doctor on preventing the illness from recurring once the child has recovered.
- Administering extended-release penicillin for three weeks to forestall relapse.
- Addressing accompanying symptoms like inflammation of the heart and joints.

Diphtheria

Diphtheria is a severe bacterial disease caused by the Corynebacterium diphtheriae bacterium. It spreads through airborne particles, direct physical contact with an infected person, or contact with contaminated objects or food. The bacteria commonly infect the nose and throat, forming a grey-to-black, tough, fiber-like covering that can obstruct the airways. Sometimes, diphtheria may initially infect the skin, resulting in skin lesions. Once infected, toxins produced by the bacteria can disseminate through the bloodstream to other organs, such as the heart, leading to substantial damage.

Incubation period

The incubation period for diphtheria ranges from one to seven days.

Symptoms of diphtheria

- Bluish coloration of the skin (cyanosis)
- Bloody, watery drainage from the nose
- Breathing problems:
- Difficulty breathing
- Rapid breathing
- Stridor (high-pitched wheezing sound)
- Chills
- Croup-like (barking) cough
- Drooling (suggesting airway blockage is imminent)
- Fever
- Hoarseness
- Painful swallowing
- Skin lesions (typically observed in tropical regions)
- Sore throat (varying from mild to severe)

Complications of diphtheria

- Inflammation of the heart muscle (myocarditis), potentially leading to heart failure.

- Inflammation of the nerves, which can result in temporary paralysis.
- Poor blood circulation, often accompanied by severe sweating, cyanosis (bluish skin), and cold extremities. This condition typically involves hyperventilation or rapid breathing.
- Inflammation of the lungs.
- Inflammation and impaired function of the kidneys.

Prevention and treatment

- Vaccination against diphtheria.
- Prompt initiation of treatment under the supervision of a doctor.
- A large dose of penicillin solution is administered via injection to the patient.
- Provide the patient with easily swallowable foods such as yogurt and juice.
- Ensuring complete rest for the patient and promptly addressing any complications.
- Complete isolation of the patient from healthy children.

CHAPTER FOURTEEN:
Accident prevention and first Aid

Keeping your child safe from accidents

Small children are particularly vulnerable to accidents because they lack an understanding of the dangers around them. For instance, they may not comprehend concepts like gravity or the harmful effects of ingesting certain substances. Unfortunately, accidents involving children are common due to parents neglecting to make their homes safe and failing to implement necessary safety measures. As soon as a child begins to crawl or walk, their natural curiosity leads them to explore and play with anything they encounter, often without recognizing the potential dangers. Therefore, parents must create a safe environment for their children. Below are some measures that can help prevent accidents:

Prevention of poisoning

Hospital emergency rooms frequently encounter cases of poisoning in children, often resulting from inadequate safety measures implemented in the home.

The most common substances that could lead to poisoning in children

- Iron supplements for treating anemia and other medications resembling candy to young children.
- Various petroleum-based products like paraffin and gasoline.
- Household insecticides.
- Laundry stain removers.
- Nail polish remover.
- Tranquilizers and contraceptive pills.
- Cigarettes.

Measures to prevent poisoning

- Store all medicines out of children's reach.
- Place insecticides and cleaning products where children cannot access them.
- Ensure medications do not resemble candy to prevent accidental ingestion.
- Keep cosmetics away from children.
- Avoid leaving cigarette packets accessible to children, as ingesting even one cigarette could be fatal for a one-year-old.
- Install locks on cabinets and drawers containing hazardous items like medicines and insecticides.

Prevention of choking and suffocation

To prevent choking or suffocation in your child:

- Store small items like coins, beads, and peanuts out of reach.
- Cut fruit into small pieces or mash it to prevent choking.
- Slice sausages lengthways instead of into round pieces.
- Keep plastic bags away from children to avoid suffocation risks.
- Ensure curtains and furnishings have no loose strings to prevent strangulation hazards.
- Choose toys without small pieces that can be swallowed and with no sharp corners.
- Keep the toilet seat closed and locked to prevent falls.
- Avoid sleeping next to your child in the same bed to prevent accidental smothering.
- Keep unused fridges and empty cupboards securely closed to prevent entrapment.
- Store gas canisters out of reach to prevent accidental opening by children.

To prevent broken bones and falls from high places:

- Keep floors dry to prevent slips and falls.
- Avoid using small rugs that can slip on tiled floors.
- Use rubber mats in the bathroom and bathtub to prevent slipping.
- Refrain from using baby walkers to reduce the risk of accidents.
- Keep tables and chairs away from windows and balconies.
- Install barriers to block access to windows and high places.
- Opt for non-slip tiles or ceramic flooring.
- Supervise children closely, especially as they start to crawl and walk, to prevent accidents.

To prevent fire and electric shock

- Keep matches and lighters locked away and out of reach of children.
- Store gas canisters securely to prevent children from playing with them.
- Protect children from gas stoves and electric heaters to avoid fire hazards.
- Cover all electrical outlets to prevent children from inserting objects.
- Have fire extinguishers in the home and know how to use them.

- Avoid carrying the child while cooking, ironing, or smoking.
- Keep hotplates, vessels, and hot irons out of reach of children and store them safely after use.
- Avoid using long tablecloths on dining tables to prevent children from pulling them and causing hot foods to spill.

First Aid for children

Disclaimer: The provided information is for informational purposes only and should not be considered a substitute for professional medical advice, emergency treatment, or formal first-aid training. It is not intended for use in diagnosing or developing a treatment plan for any health problem or disease without consulting a qualified healthcare provider. If you are in a life-threatening emergency, please seek medical assistance immediately.

First Aid for poisoning

How do I know if my child has consumed a poisonous substance?

- Sudden and severe abdominal cramps or pain without a temperature rise.
- Discovering your child with an empty bottle of medicine or any other toxic substance nearby.
- Noticing a change in color or burns in your child's mouth.
- Sudden difficulty in breathing.

- Sudden onset of nausea or vomiting.
- Increased saliva production and a change in its smell.

What to do in the event of poisoning

- Immediately take the toxic substance out of the child's hand and preserve anything that remains, including the empty bottle, to show it to the doctor. If the substance has been swallowed, remove any remnants from the mouth.
- Refrain from giving the child medicine like ipecac to induce vomiting as it may worsen the situation.
- If the child has spilled a toxic substance on their body, wear clean gloves, clean up any remaining substance from the child's body, remove their clothes, and wash their body with cool or tepid water.
- Call an ambulance or take the child to the nearest hospital for treatment.
- Bring any remnants of the toxic substance or the container to show to the doctor.

First Aid for burns

Fires pose significant risks to children, often leading to household accidents. Burns can result from exposure to flames, heat, hot liquids, or metal, as well as chemical burns or electric shocks. Burns are categorized as follows:

- First degree: characterized by redness and pain.
- Second degree: red with blisters and pain.
- Third degree: appearing stiff and white or brown.
- Fourth degree: blackened and charred, often with slough or dead tissue.

First Aid for first and second-degree burns

- Immediately cool the burn with cool (not cold) water, either by holding the affected area under a tap or immersing it in cool water. Continue for 10 to 15 minutes or until the pain subsides.
- Loosely wrap the affected part with a sterile gauze bandage or clean cloth. Avoid using fluffy cotton or materials that may leave lint in the wound.
- For burns affecting the face, eyes, or covering a large area, seek medical assistance promptly.
- Refrain from bursting or tampering with blisters, as they protect the skin from infection.

First Aid for third and fourth-degree burns

- Call an ambulance immediately.
- Avoid removing burned clothing, but ensure the victim is no longer in contact with smoldering materials, smoke, or heat.
- Refrain from immersing large severe burns in cold water to prevent hypothermia and shock.

- Check for signs of circulation such as breathing, coughing, or movement. If there are no signs, start CPR.
- Elevate the burned body part or parts, if possible, above heart level.
- Cover the burn area with a cool, damp, sterile bandage, clean cloth, or damp towels.

Chemical burns

- Remove the child's clothing.
- Gently wash the affected area with cool water.
- Wrap the area loosely with sterile gauze or clean cloth.
- Refer to the information on the container; there are often instructions on how to deal with burns caused by the substance in question.

For severe or extensive burns, burns on the eyes or face, or symptoms of shock (such as fainting, pale complexion, or shallow breathing), seek emergency medical assistance immediately.

First Aid for breaks and fractures

Broken bones are fairly common in children, particularly as they become older and more adventurous. When a bone breaks, known medically as a fracture, it necessitates medical attention. Here are some signs indicating a fracture:

- Being unable to move the affected part normally.
- Experiencing intense and unbearable pain.
- Swelling occurring at the location of the break.
- Sometimes, the sound of the fracture may be audible when it occurs. In an "open fracture," the end of the broken bone may protrude from the skin.

First Aid for a child with a fracture

- Contact emergency medical services immediately.
- If it's an open fracture, stop the bleeding.
- Refrain from moving the child if there's suspicion of a fracture in the head, neck, or back.
- Only move the child if necessary to prevent further injury.
- Provide support to the affected limb comfortably to prevent further damage and maintain the bone's position until professional assistance arrives.
- Avoid attempting to reset the bone or push any exposed bone back into place.
- Withhold food or drink until the child is evaluated by a doctor, especially if surgery requiring general anesthesia might be necessary.
- Refrain from administering painkillers until the child has been assessed by a doctor.
- Apply ice packs to alleviate swelling and pain. Without an ice pack, a bag of frozen vegetables can be used.

First Aid for near-drowning

Near drowning occurs when someone survives a drowning incident but experiences unconsciousness or inhales water. It can happen to a child who falls into a swimming pool, bathtub, or from your arms at the beach. If this happens, take these steps immediately:

- Call for an ambulance.
- Administer CPR if the child has lost consciousness, lacks a pulse, and/or is not breathing.
- Remove wet clothing and cover the child with blankets to prevent hypothermia.

First Aid for wounds and bleeding

Minor cuts and scrapes are common in childhood and often don't require medical attention. Here's what to do when dealing with such injuries:

- Stop bleeding by applying pressure to the wound with gauze or a clean cloth.
- Clean the wound with surgical spirits or rubbing alcohol.
- Use tweezers (cleaned with rubbing alcohol) to remove small debris. Larger or deeply embedded debris should be removed by a doctor.
- Apply a topical antiseptic like Neosporin or Polysporin to prevent infection.

- Cover the wound with a clean dressing or band-aid. Ensure the gauze pad fully covers the wound.
- If bleeding persists and seeps through the dressing, apply another dressing.
- Seek medical attention if the wound is large and may require stitches.

First Aid for bites and stings Animal bites

- An animal bite can transmit diseases or infections, especially if rabies is risky. Seek medical help immediately; immunization can prevent infection if administered promptly.
- Allow some bleeding to cleanse the wound, but apply pressure to control severe bleeding.
- Wash the wound with antiseptic soap and cover it with a dressing.

Snake bites

If you reside where venomous snakes are present, educate your child about snake awareness and advise them not to disturb or attempt to handle them. If a snake bite occurs, follow these steps:

- Keep the affected limb below the level of the heart.
- Apply a constricting band to slow the spread of poison: place the band between the bite and the heart, approximately 5-10 cm above the wound.

Ensure it's not too tight; you should be able to slide two fingers underneath.

It's not recommended to attempt to suck the poison out or to cut the skin where the bite occurred.

Insect bites and stings

Most insect bites and stings typically result in a few days of itching and mild swelling, which can be uncomfortable for your child but are generally not serious. For mild cases like these, consider the following steps:

- Reassure and comfort your child.
- Remove the stinger, especially if embedded in the skin, to prevent further venom release.
- Wash the affected area with soap and water.
- Apply an ice pack to reduce pain and swelling.
- Administer hydrocortisone cream, calamine lotion, or a baking soda paste to the bite or sting several times daily until symptoms improve.
- Provide your child with an antihistamine containing diphenhydramine (Benadryl, Tylenol Severe Allergy) or chlorpheniramine maleate (Chlor-Trimeton, Actifed).
- Watch out for delayed reactions such as fever, hives, joint pain, or swollen glands. If these occur, seek medical attention promptly.

In some cases, children with allergies to bee or wasp stings may experience severe anaphylaxis, characterized by symptoms such as nausea, facial swelling, difficulty breathing, faintness, abdominal pain, rapid heartbeat, or shock. This constitutes a medical emergency; immediately call for an ambulance. If your child has a known allergy and has been prescribed an epinephrine auto-injector, ensure you and others around your child know how to use it.

First Aid for eye injuries

The child might encounter a foreign object in their eye, such as a small flying insect, dust, or sand. In such cases:

- Gently pull the lower eyelid out and look for the foreign object. If it's not visible, gently lift the upper eyelid until you locate it.
- Carefully remove the foreign body using the corner of a wet tissue or clean, lint-free cloth.
- Rinse the child's eye with water until the foreign object is completely eliminated.
- If the foreign object remains and the eye is still red and swollen, seek medical attention.
- If you cannot remove the object or if it's embedded in the eyeball, seek immediate medical assistance.

These scenarios highlight a few instances where a child may require first Aid. Parents must learn first-aid techniques and be prepared to respond to emergencies before they occur. First aid courses are available in many areas, and online resources provide ample information for further learning.

www.ingramcontent.com/pod-product-compliance
Lightning Source LLC
Chambersburg PA
CBHW051549250726

48653CB00004BA/1055